Essentials of
Local Anesthesia
with MCQs

Essentials of Local Anesthesia with MCQs

KG Ghorpade
MDS
Principal
Professor and Head
Oral and Maxillofacial Surgery Dept.
Sri Venkateshwara Dental College and Hospital
Bangalore (INDIA)

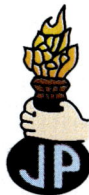

JAYPEE BROTHERS
MEDICAL PUBLISHERS (P) LTD
New Delhi

Published by

Jitendar P Vij

Jaypee Brothers Medical Publishers (P) Ltd

EMCA House, 23/23B Ansari Road, Daryaganj

New Delhi 110 002, India

Phones: +91-11-23272143, +91-11-23272703, +91-11-23282021, +91-11-23245672

Fax: +91-11-23276490, +91-11-23245683   e-mail: jaypee@jaypeebrothers.com

Visit our website: www.jaypeebrothers.com

Branches

- 2/B, Akruti Society, Jodhpur Gam Road Satellite
  Ahmedabad 380015,   Phone: +91-079-30988717

- 202 Batavia Chambers, 8 Kumara Krupa Road, Kumara Park East
  Bangalore 560 001, Phones: +91-80-22285971, +91-80-22382956, +91-80-30614073
  Tele Fax: +91-80-22281761   e-mail: jaypeemedpubbgl@eth.net

- 282 IIIrd Floor, Khaleel Shirazi Estate, Fountain Plaza
  Pantheon Road, **Chennai** 600 008, Phones: +91-44-28262665, +91-44-28269897
  Fax: +91-44-28262331   e-mail: jpchen@eth.net

- 4-2-1067/1-3, Ist Floor, Balaji Building, Ramkote
  Cross Road, **Hyderabad** 500 095, Phones: +91-40-55610020, +91-40-24758498
  Fax: +91-40-24758499   e-mail: jpmedpub@rediffmail.com

- 1A Indian Mirror Street, Wellington Square
  Kolkata 700 013, Phones: +91-33-22456075, +91-33-22451926
  Fax: +91-33-22456075   e-mail: jpbcal@cal.vsnl.net.in

- 106 Amit Industrial Estate, 61 Dr SS Rao Road, Near MGM Hospital
  Parel, **Mumbai** 400 012, Phones: +91-22-24124863, +91-22-24104532,
  +91-22-30926896 Fax: +91-22-24160828   e-mail: jpmedpub@bom7.vsnl.net.in

- "KAMALPUSHPA" 38, Reshimbag Opp Mohota Science College,
  Umred Road, **Nagpur** 440 009 (MS), Phone: +91-712-3945220, +91-712-2704275
  e-mail: jpmednagpur@rediffmail.com

Essentials of Local Anesthesia with MCQs

First Edition: **2006**

ISBN 81-8061-735-1

Typeset at JPBMP typesetting unit
Printed at Sanat Printers, Kundli.

With great pleasure I dedicate this book to

my ever encouraging wife

SHASHI

and to my loving children

SHUMAL and KAUSHAL

Preface

The practice of dentistry has undergone tremendous changes over the past three decades. Appearance of newer diseases has triggered improvements in patient handling, sterilization methods, better understanding of drug action, managing complications and personal protection. In todays modern practice local anesthesia plays an important role. Every speciality in dentistry employs local anesthesia in one way or the other. Without the knowledge of effective administration of local anesthetics, it is not possible for any dental surgeon to deliver satisfactory and qualitative treatment.

This book on local anesthesia has been written in view of the requirements of undergraduate and postgraduate students especially in Indian context. The book covers basics of Pharmacology of local anesthetic drugs, anatomy, neurophysiology, mechanism of action of local anesthetic, varied techniques in administration of local anesthesia, complications and their management. All the latest developments and anesthetic products and the drug delivery system has been included. The products available in India and the armamentarium used has been emphasized. Detailed techniques of drug administration and management of complications of local anesthesia has been elaborated. This is the first book on local anesthesia by an Indian author. The text has been prepared in easy style to understand language. Numerous diagrams, illustrations which are schematic have been included to enhance understanding of the subject. To make a few controversies better understood, certain details have been omitted. Students should find the book interesting to read and with the help of diagrams and photographs understand the subject matter easily.

This book serves the needs of all dental students and dental practitioners. For postgraduates it should serve as a basis of local anesthesia with reference to other books.

Most of the competitive and entrance examinations in India follow the multiple choice questions. This is an excellent trend as the students can be assessed in all the chapters in a particular subject. Keeping this in view a chapter on multiple choice questions has been included to benefit the students.

An attempt has been made to bring out a comprehensive textbook on local anesthesia and will be glad if the dental students and fraternity find it useful.

KG Ghorpade

Acknowledgements

I owe special debt of gratitude for the expert help of Dr A Sreenivasa Babu, Chief Consultant Anesthesiologist, Department of Anesthesiology and Intensive Care, The Bangalore Hospital, Bangalore with section on premedication and sedation techniques.

I am extremely grateful to Dr Vinutha Shankar, Professor of Physiology for her suggestions and help with section on Physiology and Neuroanatomy.

I would like to extend my special thanks to Dr Harinarayan Rao, Professor of Surgery and Dr Bharat for their invaluable help in preparation of excellent photographs.

It is only the encouragement and support from Jaypee Brothers Medical Publishers which made it possible for me to write this book. I thank all the help rendered by the staff of Bangalore office.

My special thanks goes to Mr. Hasan Mansoor, former Professor of English for his kind help in editing the manuscript.

I would be failing in my duty if I do not acknowledge the whole hearted help from M/s Astra – Zeneca, Bangalore, India, Warren Pharmaceuticals, Group Pharmaceuticals and Muller and Phipps (India).

I am highly thankful to Dr Rashmi Thitte, Dr Seema Gowda, Dr Kumara Swamy, Dr Sridhar, Dr Prasanna and Dr Bipin for their assistance in preparation of this book.

My sincere gratitude to Mr Kiran Kumar and Mr. Dattatreya of Dream team for their great help in preparation of diagrams and CD's.

I gratefully acknowledge Dr Palak Pandya, Dr Nandini, Dr Madhura, Dr Saurav Chowdhury and Mr Chetan for their cooperation and patience during photo sessions.

Last but not the least, I gratefully acknowledge the kind help of Miss Varalakshmi for the secretarial help in preparation of this manuscript.

SPECIAL NOTE

I would like to first thank my parents, my brothers and the entire Ghorpade family without whose help I would not have been where I am today.

Contents

1

Pharmacology of Local Anesthetics

HISTORY OF DEVELOPMENT OF LOCAL ANESTHESIA

Pain has been in existence ever since human being came into this world. Dental pain is considered to be the worst amongst pain due to ailments. It is but natural to acclaim the discovery of drugs, which controlled pain during dental procedures. The only method available a century ago in control of pain was the use of opium and alcohol. It is worthwhile to read a few lines about those great people who heralded the development of the local anesthesia.

It was in 1842 that, a physician named Crawford Long used ether to cause euphoria, under the influence of which a minor surgery was performed. Although Horace Wells was the one who in 1844 demonstrated the properties of nitrous oxide. It was Joseph Priestly who first brought to notice, the effect of N_2O. Horace Wells got one of his own tooth removed under the influence of N_2O and it was without any pain!.

In Pre-Columbian times, natives in South America used leaves of coca a local shrub (erythroxylon coca) for mystical, religious, social, nutritional and medical purposes. By chewing the leaves of coca, the natives found it gave them relief from hunger and fatigue. In 1551, use of coca leaves was banned but the invaders later found that without chewing of the leaves, the workers could hardly work in the fields or mine gold. Since it enhanced endurance and promoted a sense of well-being it was distributed three or four times a day to the workers during brief period of rest. These leaves were brought to

Europe to extract the active principle. After much experimenting, Gaedicke in 1855 isolated the alkaloid erythroxylin from the coca leaves. Albert Niemann a chemist in 1860 was successful in isolating cocaine from erythroxylin. In the year 1879 von Anrep found that diluted solution of cocaine when injected caused the skin to become numb and the pupils dilated when the solution was dropped on the eye. Sigmund Freud studied the properties of cocaine and wrote a paper highlighting the properties of cocaine. Carl Koller hearing the comments of Dr. Engel about the numbing effect of the crystals of cocaine on tongue hastened to experiment with diluted solution of cocaine on the cornea of his own eye. He was excited about its anesthetic effect and in the same year (1884) demonstrated the effectiveness of cocaine on mucous membrane at a conference in Vienna. Thus Koller heralded the use of cocaine as an anesthetic agent. Finally it was William Halstead who in 1885 administered the first inferior alveolar nerve block using 4% cocaine in solution. Although the cocaine's benefits became popular the toxic and habit-forming properties surfaced. Many fatalities were reported a few years after its introduction. In spite of these disadvantages, cocaine was widely used for nearly 10 years.

Willstatter and associates in 1895 explained the chemical structure, the benzoic acid methyl ester, which initiated further research in benzoic acid esters. Although many synthetic compounds with anesthetic properties were introduced, they were unable to replace cocaine.

Meanwhile Einhorn after number of years of experimenting with many compounds succeeded in synthesizing procaine in 1904. This local anesthetic was less toxic and importantly was not addictive. Procaine became the choice of local anesthetic for the next 40 years.

Erdman, right from 1940 was experimenting with alkaloid gramine and was surprised to find the numbing effect of the drug on the tongue. Probably tasting the chemicals was a way of determining some properties of any chemical. It was Lófgren in 1943 who continued the research work and successfully synthesized lidocaine, an aniline derivative. This heralded a new era of non-toxic anesthetic agent. Lidocaine is being used even today and has found general acceptance as a safe and effective local anesthetic drug. Since then many more anesthetic agents have been developed, some having rapid onset and some showing long duration of action. The research still continues for an ideal anesthetic agent.

DESIRED PROPERTIES OF AN IDEAL ANESTHETIC AGENT

1. The action of an anesthetic agent should be reversible.

   During any dental procedure the purpose of an anesthetic agent is to ensure that the patient does not feel any sensation of pain. The anesthetic effect should be in the teeth and the surrounding supporting structures. After a short duration of time, normal sensation should return in the area of anesthesia.

2. The anesthetic solution should be compatible with the tissue fluids.

   The anesthetic solution is usually injected into the tissues in the area of nerve distribution. The solution so injected should not act as an irritant to the tissues. The patient should feel comfortable during the deposition, and its absorption.

3. Onset of action of the anesthetic agent should be rapid.

   Rapid effect of the anesthetic solution in the area is important since neither the patient nor the dental surgeon need to wait for the continuation of treatment. If the waiting period is prolonged before onset of anesthesia the patient may become more apprehensive.

4. The duration of action should be sufficient for varying procedures.

   The majority of dental procedures undertaken in general dentistry usually lasts from 10 minutes to 30 minutes. If the anesthesia lasts more than 30 minutes the patient is left to wait with the uncomfortable feeling of numbness. Apart from the uncomfortable feeling, the patient may injure his or her lips or check by accidental biting.

5. The anesthetic solution should possess rapid diffusion property.

   The anesthetic solution when injected in the vicinity of the nerve branches, should diffuse up to the nerve in the shortest possible time. It should be able to diffuse through the periosteum, bone and interstitial tissue. This property of diffusion will minimize the number of needle penetration made during infiltration anesthesia.

6. It should possess low systemic toxicity.

   All anesthetic agents cause certain amount of excitation and stimulation of central nervous system (CNS) and cardiovascular system. In cases of excess dosage it may result in undesirable effects. Toxicity depends upon the absorption, percentage of anesthetic in circulation and the rate of excretion from the body. An ideal anesthetic should be clinically active in low concentration and possess low toxicity.

7. There should be rapid excretion from the body.

   This depends upon the hydrolysis of the drug in the blood, liver and excretion in the kidneys. When there is rapid excretion, the anesthetic agent is removed from the circulation and symptoms of toxicity may not be seen.

8. Should be able to achieve maximum anesthetic effect with minimum amount of dosage.

   The anesthetic agent should be potent even in low dosage. This depends upon the protein binding property of the particular anesthetic agent, presence of a vasoconstrictor, technique of administration and the vascularity of the area.

9. It should be free of allergic reactions.

Certain anesthetic agents cause allergy, which sometimes could be severe. Apart from anesthetic agents, constituents like vasoconstrictor and preservatives may cause allergic reactions. The amide group of anesthetic drugs do not cause any allergic reactions but preservatives used in anesthetic solution may cause allergic reactions.

10. It should be stable in solution form with a long shelf life.

The anesthetic base which are unstable are combined with strong acid to make them stable. When vasoconstrictors are used, preservatives and antioxidizing agents are added to increase the shelf life.

11. It should not be a habit-forming drug.

Cocaine, which was being used as an anesthetic agent resulted in habit formation. The preparations available at present are free from addiction.

12. It should be compatible with other constituents in the anesthetic solution. Many constituents like preservatives, antifungal agents, antiseptics and vasoconstrictors are added to the anesthetic solution to achieve certain desirable properties as the anesthetic agent by itself may not be ideal. These constituents when added together should be compatible with each other and should not intereact and cause undesirable effects.

LOCAL ANESTHESIA—TERMINOLOGY

General anesthesia refers to loss of consciousness and the action is on central nervous system. In local anesthesia the action is on peripheral nerves and the patient will be awake. The term analgesia is applied when there is loss of pain sensation alone. Local anesthesia causes loss of pain, pressure, touch and temperature in a localized area. In many of the dental procedures local dental analgesia could be ideal and comfortable, however it will not be

possible to achieve selective analgesia by the use of anesthetic drugs. Local anesthesia can be achieved by the following methods:

1. By reducing the temperature of the area (e.g. spraying of ethyl chloride).
2. Selective sectioning of nerve fibers.
3. Permanent or long term loss of sensation by application of chemicals.
4. Use of drugs to temporarily stop transmission of nerve impulses.

In this book the discussion is restricted to use of local anesthetic drugs in control of pain.

CHEMISTRY

Chemically, all anesthetic agents consist of an anesthetic portion, a linkage chain and a secondary or tertiary amino group. Local anesthetic drugs are synthesized by linking various chemical groups to the aromatic portion and the amino groups. The chemical could be an ester or of amide linkage (Fig. 1-1). The drugs thus synthesized are in general viscid liquids or amorphous solids. These components are usually in basic form and are not soluble in water. Hence they are combined with a strong acid to form hydrochloride which is soluble in water (Fig. 1-2).

Fig. 1-1: General molecular configuration

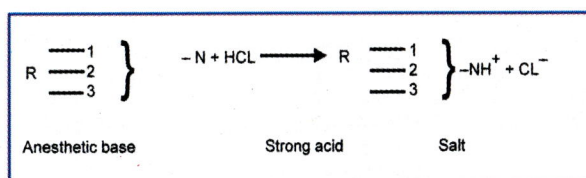

Fig.1-2: Formation of an hydrochloride salt

All the anesthetics preparations are in acidic form and are stable. In the acidic state, the anesthetics are almost completely in ionized state. It is essential that nonionized free base is required for penetration of lipid membranous nerve tissue. When the anesthetic solution is deposited in the tissues, the abundant tissue fluid which is in basic state dilutes the acidic anesthetic solution to basic state. By this action certain percentage of free base is liberated which is in non-ionized form and will be available for penetration of the nerve membrane. It is important to note that ionized form of the anesthetic drug is also required for blocking the conduction of nerve impulses. The percentage of ionized and non-ionized parts depends upon the surrounding liquid pH and dissociation constant (pKa – is approximate by equal proportion of ionic and non-ionic form present in the anesthetic solution which is constant for each anesthetic drug) of the anesthetic drug used (Fig. 1-3). On entering the nerve cell through the cell membrane the non-ionized form dissociates to ionic form and binds with protein in sodium channel. This blocks the sodium infusion and thus the transmission of nerve impulse is blocked (Fig. 1-4).

The percentage of unionized form is higher in amide group of drugs when compared with ester group of drugs. This results in quicker penetration of the nerve membrane and early onset of action. The binding of the ionized form with plasma proteins is a reversible process. When the binding is prolonged the action of the anesthetics lasts longer.

Absorption, Metabolism and Excretion

When the anesthetic solution is injected into tissues it spreads in all directions. Part of the solution infiltrates

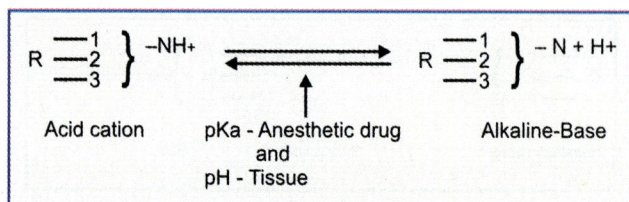

Fig.1-3: Cation-Base ratio

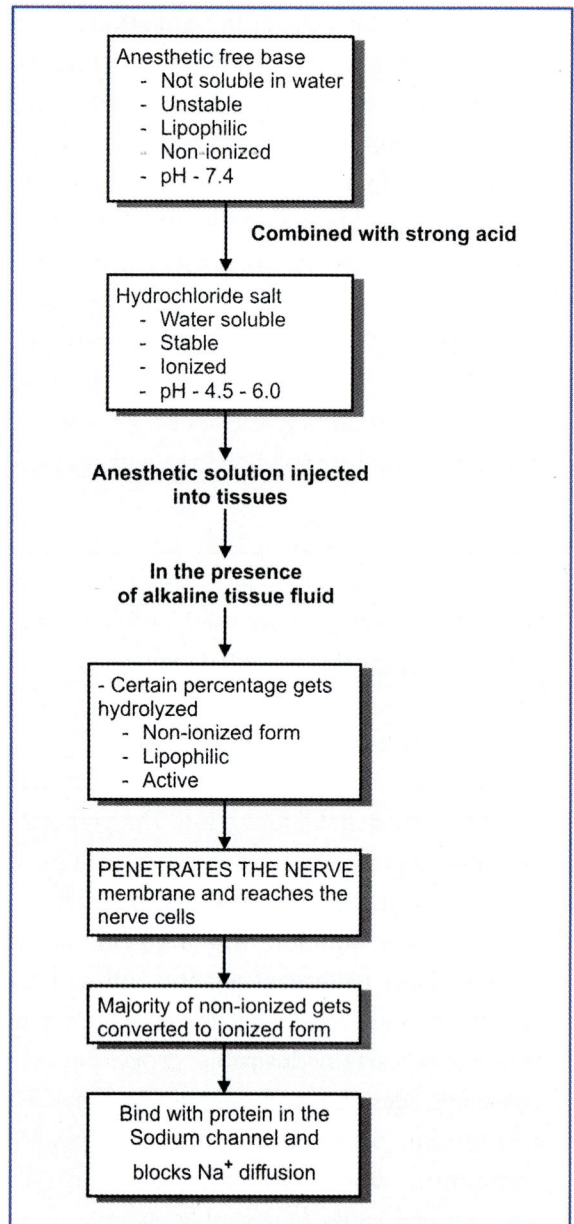

Fig.1-4: Steps in action of local anesthetic drug

the nerve tissue and part of it gets absorbed into circulation. Once the action of the anesthetic solution on the nerve tissue wears away it is slowly absorbed into circulation. The amount of solution which enters the circulation depends on:

1. The vascularity of the area into which the anesthetic solution has been deposited—Higher the vascularity higher is concentration of anesthetic solution entering the circulation.

2. Presence of a vasoconstrictor in the anesthetic solution—If there is no vasoconstrictor in the anesthetic solution then the solution is quickly absorbed into circulation. If there is a vasoconstrictor then there is slow absorption of the anesthetic solution and its presence in the tissues is prolonged.

3. The protein binding properties of the anesthetic solution—If the protein binding is prolonged, there is longer lasting anesthesia; at the same time there is slow absorption of part of the anesthetic solution.

As the absorbed anesthetic solution enters the blood, circulation it is distributed to all the parts of the body. The anatomical parts which are highly vascular attract more of anesthetic drug. Central nervous system, lungs, liver, kidney and spleen absorb major portion of the anesthetic solution. The circulating drug gets hydrolyzed in plasma, liver and is excreted through kidneys. Certain percentage of anesthetic drug is excreted through kidney in free form.

Most of the anesthetic agents used belong either to ester groups or to amide group of drugs. In case of ester groups, major portion of the drug is hydrolyzed in the blood plasma within a short period. Pseudocholinesterase present in the plasma converts the drug into para-amino benzoic acid (PABA). The metabolite PABA causes the allergic reaction related to procaine. The metabolites and the unchanged drug are excreted through kidneys.

The amide group of anesthetics is metabolized primarily in the liver, however prilocaine, undergoes certain amount of biotransformation in the lungs. The biotransformation of the amide group take much more time than the ester group. Administration of amide group of anesthetics in the patients suffering from liver diseases should be dealt with caution. In elderly patients due to reduced function of the liver, dosage of the anesthetic solution should be reduced to prevent toxic effects. As in case of ester group of drugs the end products are excreted through kidneys.

Cocaine

Cocaine is derived from leaves of coca plant. It was used as a local anesthetic for a long period of time. Although it has been used for block anesthesia in the form of anesthetic solution, it is more effective as a surface anesthetic. The drug is highly toxic and habit-forming. Overdosage of the drug results in tremors, convulsions, myocardial depression and death may result due to respiratory failure. At present, cocaine is not used in dental practice since better and safer local anesthetics are available.

Derivatives of Ester Group of Anesthetics

Procaine Hydrochloride (Novocaine, Bayer)

Procaine hydrochloride was synthesized from para-amino benzoic acid in 1904 by Einhorn. The anesthetic proved to be very useful in dental local anesthesia. Procaine is diethyl amino-ethyl ester. The hydrochloride form is water soluble and successfully used for infiltration and block anesthesia. It is not very useful as a surface anesthetic, since its absorption from the surface is poor. Procaine has a vasodilatory action and hence is absorbed quickly from the site of deposition. Adrenaline, in the ratio of 1:50,000 or 1:100,000 is added to the anesthetic solution, which causes vasoconstriction of the blood vessels in the local area and thereby delays the absorption of the anesthetic solution. The anesthetic effect approximately lasts for 2 hours. Procaine is hydrolyzed in the blood by pseudocholinesterase and is in turn excreted through the kidneys. Procaine can sensitize patients and cause allergic reactions.

Other Ester Group of Anesthetic Agents

Amethocaine(Tetracaine)
• Used in 0.5 to 2% concentration
• More useful as surface anesthetic
• Not suitable for injections
• More toxic than procaine.

Tetracaine (Pontocaine)
- Used in 2% solution
- More useful as surface anesthetic
- Slow onset and longer duration of action
- Less toxic than procaine.

Propoxycaine (Rovacaine)
- Less potent and less toxic than procaine.
- Used in combination with procaine 4% Propoxycaine with 2% Procaine and leverternol in 1: 30,000
- Rapid onset of action.

2 Chlorprocaine (Nesacaine)
- Used in 2% solution
- Potent analgesic
- Increased toxicity
- Short duration of action
- Not a reliable local anesthetic.

Meta Amino Benzoic Acid Esters Derivatives

Metabutethamine (Unacaine)
- Less toxic than procaine
- Short acting
- Rapid onset of action.

Metabutoxycaine (Primacaine)
- Less toxic than procaine
- Longer duration of action.

Benzoic Acid Ester Derivatives

- Piperocaine (Metycaine)—Similar action as procaine.
- Meprylcaine (Oracaine)—Faster onset of action.
- Isobucaine (Kincaine)—Longer duration of action.

Anilide Non-ester Group

Lignocaine

Anilide non-ester group of drugs are extensively used in Dentistry. The most important advantage of this group of drugs is that they contain amide linkage which does not sensitize the patients unlike ester group of drugs. The amide group of drugs are more potent and equally toxic. The first form of anesthetic from this group was lignocaine

and was synthesized by Nil Lofgren in 1943. Since that time it has become most popular and widely used anesthetic drug in Dentistry. It is used as a hydrochloride salt and is equally effective both for injections and surface anesthesia. The drug is used in 2% solution and since it has a vasodilatory effect it is rapidly absorbed into the blood stream. To retain the solution in the local area, vasoconstrictors are added which reduces rapid absorption and prevents chances of toxicity. Although the maximum total dosage is 25 ml of 2% solution (500 mg) with adrenaline, 15 ml of solution can be safely used in healthy patients. In most instances, for any procedure performed in dental office, a dentist rarely uses more than 6 to 8 ml of anesthetic agent. This gives a high safety margin. The lignocaine is hydrolyzed in liver, which is then excreted along with part of unchanged drug through kidneys. Lignocaine in medical practice is used in the dosage of 60 to 100 mg i.v. to correct ventricular arrhythmias.

In large doses the drug has a depressive action on the myocardium. Majority of the anesthetic drugs cause initial excitation of CNS but in case of Lidocaine the first reaction to overdosage is that of depression which is clinically noticed as feeling sleepy by the patients.

Mepivacaine (Carbocaine, Isocaine, Arestocaine)

Mepivacaine, a derivative of xylidine was introduced in 1960. This drug has a similar action as lignocaine and is used in 2% solution with 1:80,000 adrenaline. Although the action is similar to lignocaine its action is shorter compared to lignocaine. As mepivocaine has a diminished vasodilatory effect, it can be used without a vasoconstrictor in 3% solution. Without vasoconstrictor the drug has a long shelf life. For 2% solution with vasoconstrictor, the maximum dosage should be 300 mg or 15 ml. Mepivocaine is less toxic compared to lignocaine but is not useful as a topical anesthetic.

Bupivocaine (Monocaine)

This is a derivative of amide group and is four times more potent than lignocaine. It has a slow rate of onset and the anesthetic effect lasts for a longer duration. Bupivocaine can be used in minor oral surgical procedures lasting more than 1½ hrs. Due to its longer duration of action the postoperative pain is also controlled. It has a vasodilatory action on blood vessels and hence should be used along with a vasoconstrictor. It is used in 0.5% solution with 1:200,000 epinephrine. Its use in pregnant women is contraindicated since it may cause cardiac complications in cases of accidental intravenous injections.

Prilocaine (Citanest)

Prilocaine differs from lidocaine in that it is a toluidine derivative. It is the most recent anesthetic agent introduced from the amide group. Prilocaine is less potent and less toxic. It has a prolonged action. The diminished toxic effect may be due to its rapid metabolism in the liver. Large doses of prilocaine can result in methemoglobinemia. It is contraindicated in children and pregnant women. The drug is metabolized in liver and lungs. It is used in 4% solution with 1:200,000 epinephrine.

Etidocaine (Durannt)

Etidocaine is a derivative of amide group and its action resembles that of lidocaine, and is used in 1.5% solution with 1:200,000 epinephrine. The duration of action is more compared to lidocaine.

Butamilicaine Phosphate (Hostacain)

This is derived from amide group and has a similar action compared to lignocaine except that the vasodilatory effect is less. It is used in combination with 1% procaine (Hostacain SP). The availability is 2% solution with 1:50,000 adrenaline. Hostacain NOR 2% solution with non-adrenaline in 1:25,000 concentration is also used. Hostacain SP has a longer duration of action than Hostacain NOR. Both these preparations were available in India for some time but later were withdrawn from the market.

Articaine HCL

Articaine is an amide derivative introduced in Europe in 1976. Its use in USA was approved in the year 2000. This drug preparation is not available in India. Articaine although an amide derivative also contains an ester component. Articaine is 1.5 times more potent than Lidocaine. It has vasodilatory action like other amide group of drugs. The onset on action of Articaine is faster and gets quickly excreted.

It is available in 4% solution with 1:100,000 and 1:200,000 adrenaline. The advantage of this drug is its supposedly excellent infiltrating properties. It is claimed that all the teeth could be anesthetized by infiltration alone. As infiltration anesthesia is the safest method of administration of local anesthesia, this drug Articaine may prove to be highly valuable.

Centbucridine

This anesthetic drug is a quinoline derivative and has been found to be as effective as lignocaine. It has been extensively tried as a local anesthetic in India. The drug has no serious side effects and no adverse effect on cardiovascular system. Even when overdose is attained there has been no untoward effect on CNS. The effect on CNS is stimulation and no depression has been noticed.

Diphenhydramine

Diphenhydramine an antihistaminic agent has been used as an effective local anesthetic in patients who are allergic to regular anesthetic drugs. The onset of action is faster but at the same time the effect lasts for a shorter duration. Control of pain is not very profound as in other anesthetic drugs but all minor procedures can be effectively managed.

Anesthetic Drugs for Topical Use

Many anesthetic agents are not water soluble and as such cannot be used for injections into the tissues. These agents when mixed with alcohol or glycol act as excellent surface anesthetics. When such preparations are applied over mucous membrane they readily penetrate the mucous membrane and anesthetize the terminal nerve endings. This results in surface anesthesia and the initial needle penetration becomes painless. To be effective, the topical anesthetic agents have to be dispensed in higher concentration. They are available in gelly, ointment, viscous liquid and spray form. Since there are no added vasoconstrictors, the anesthetic drugs get quickly absorbed into circulation. If one is not cautious this may lead to toxic levels in the blood. Surface anesthetics are not effective on skin surface.

Benzocaine

This is an ester of para-amino benzoic acid. As it is not water-soluble it is not suitable for injections. However preparations of benzocaine act as excellent surface anesthetics when applied over any type of mucous membrane. This ester group of drugs due to its poor absorption, does not cause toxicity due to overdosage. It is dispensed, as gel, gel patch and in spray form.

Lidocaine

Lidocaine can be used for both surface application and injections. For surface anesthesia the free base form of lidocaine which is not soluble in water, can be used. For injections the water soluble hydrochloride salt is used. It is available in the form of gelly (2%), topical solution (4%), ointment (5%), viscous liquid (2%) and aerosal spray (10%). Since no vasoconstrictors are added it may get quickly absorbed into circulation and result in toxic reactions. It should be used in moderate dosage.

Dyclomine

This is a ketone derivative and differs from other anesthetic agents. Its systemic absorption is poor as it is not water soluble. Onset of action is slow but the effect lasts for a longer duration. It is dispensed in 0.5% solution.

Cocaine

This naturally occurring substance is an excellent surface anesthetic. Although this drug has been used for injections for number of years it is not suitable due to its high toxic effects and habit-forming properties. Although the anesthetic agents in general are vasodilators, cocaine causes vasoconstriction. It has a quick onset and longer duration of action. As safer drugs are available, this is not being used in dentistry.

Eutectic Mixture of Local Anesthetic (EMLA)

A combination of 2.5% lidocaine and 2.5% prilocaine, EMLA is dispensed in cream form. EMLA when applied to surface of the skin, produces effective surface anesthesia. As there is slow penetration, it has to be applied one hour before the procedure. It is occluded over the skin under a dressing. The anesthetic effect lasts 2 to 3 hours. Although EMLA is mainly indicated for extraoral use it has also been found to be effective intraorally. In dentistry loose teeth extraction and minor surgery in children can be done with the use EMLA.

Vasoconstrictors

Vasoconstrictors are added to local anesthetic solution in order to:
1. Delay the absorption of the anesthetic drug from the site of deposition so that the anesthetic effect can be prolonged.
2. Reduce the rapidity of absorption in order to prevent accumulation of the drug in the blood circulation to toxic levels.
3. Control bleeding in the area of surgery.

The above factors depend upon the vascularity of the area where the solution is deposited. As the mucosal tissue in the oral cavity has abundant vascularity, the addition of vasoconstrictor is beneficial. The concentration of the vasoconstrictor used depends upon the potency and toxicity of the drug. For dental use, concentration of epinephrine varies between 1:50,000 and 1:200,000. It has been observed that 1:100,000 concentration is sufficient for effective duration of anesthesia and also to reduce toxicity.

Use of anesthetic solution with vasoconstrictor in patients with cardiovascular disease was thought to cause an increase in blood pressure which the patient may not tolerate. The amount of vasoconstrictor used in local anesthetic solution is so low that its effect on cardio-vascular system is negligible. This has been confirmed by many authors who have opined that careful injection of 2% solution after aspiration should not cause untoward action on the cardiovascular system. It is interesting to note that in a patient under anxiety and stress, there is an equal amount of adrenaline released into circulation endogenously. What is required in cardiovascular patients is careful premedication and prevention of intravascular injection while administering local anesthesia. As a guideline, the 'New York Heart Association' recommends that in one session not more than 0.2 mg of epinephrine should be administered in a healthy adult. This amounts to 10 ml of anesthetic solution with 1:50,000 adrenaline or 20 ml with 1:100,000 adrenaline. A patient with organic heart, should not receive more than 0.04 mg of epinephrine.

Adrenaline (Epinephrine)

Adrenaline is released from adrenal medulla and can be extracted from mammalian adrenaline glands or it can be synthetically manufactured. There are two types of adrenergic receptor namely, alpha and beta-receptors. Alpha receptors are related to excitary effect and beta-receptors are related to inhibitory action. Adrenaline acts on both the receptors, which results in dilatation of blood vessels in skeletal muscles and myocardium, while the vessels in skin and mucous membrane are constricted. The effect on myocardium is increase in heart rate and cardiac output. Epinephrine interacts with tricyclic antidepressant drugs and hence its use in such patients may be avoided. Local anesthetic with vasoconstrictor is sometimes used for infiltration during surgery under general anesthesia to reduce the bleeding in the area of surgical incision. General anesthetics like cyclopropane,

ethyl chloride and halothane sensitizes myocardium in the presence of adrenaline and results in ventricular fibrillations. Hence, such infiltrations should always be done with the approval of the anesthetist. To reduce such complications, anesthetic agents with vasoconstrictor felypressine can be used.

Noradrenaline (Levarterenol)

Noradrenaline is basically released by sympathetic postganglionic neurons and also to a small extent from adrenal medulla. It has a vasoconstrictor effect on vessels of skin and mucous membrane resulting in peripheral resistance. Its vasoconstrictor effect is comparatively less than epinephrine, although the effect lasts for longer duration. Toxic effects are similar to epinephrine except that norepinephrine causes severe hypertension. It is used in anesthetic solution in the concentration of 1:80,000 to 1:25,000.

Nordefin (Cobefrin) and Phenylephrine (Neophryn)

These are other sympathomimetic drugs which have vasoconstrictor action similar to that of adrenaline. The adverse reaction of adrenaline on cardia is not seen when the above two drugs are used. Its vasoconstrictor effect is less compared to adrenaline, while the toxic effects are same as that of adrenaline.

The other drugs that can be used apart from sympa-thomimetic amines as vasoconstrictor are hormones of posterior lobe of pituitary which are vasopressin, fellypressin (phenyl pressine, octapressin) and ormipressin. Vasopressin is a natural hormone whereas fellypressin and ormipressin are synthetic preparations. These preparations have similar action as that of adrenaline except that they are slow in onset of action and have prolonged effect. They can be safely used for infiltration during general anesthesia without the risk of ventricular fibrillation. They can also be safely used when tricyclic drugs are being used. They are contraindicated in pregnant women as it may cause hypoxia of placental circulation. Prilocaine 3% with fellypressin in the concentration of 0.03 per ml i.v has been successfully used in dental practice. Its safety margin in cardiac patients is quite high and hence can be safely used in such patients.

CONSTITUENTS OF LOCAL ANESTHETIC SOLUTION

1. Anesthetic base
2. Vasoconstrictors (may or may not be present)
3. Reducing agents
4. Preservative
5. Antifungal agent
6. Vehicle

1. Local anesthetic compound in basic form is unstable and is not water soluble, but in basic form it is highly lipophilic and thus can quickly penetrate the nerve tissue. Since the free base is unstable, it is combined with a strong acid to obtain a hydrochloride salt which is soluble in water. In solution form, the pH of the anesthetic drug is marginally acidic and is stable. Addition of a vasoconstrictor to the anesthetic solution makes it more acidic. When the anesthetic solution is injected into tissues the abundant interstial tissue fluid, which is normally basic in nature, hydrolyzes the small volume of anesthetic solution and the free base gets liberated. For the free base to be quickly available, the pKa of the anesthetic drug should be lower and pH of the solution higher. pKa is approximate by equal proportion of ionic and nonionic form present in the anesthetic solution which is constant for each anesthetic drug. Local anesthetic is not effective in inflamed and infected region as the tissue fluid in that region is slightly acidic. This results in ineffective hydrolysis of the anesthetic solution.

2. Vasoconstrictors—Addition of vasoconstrictors and their action has already been discussed. In some preparations, vasoconstrictors are not added and the anesthetic drug is used as plain solution. When plain anesthetic solution is used there will be quick absorption and short duration of action. Chances of overdosage should be kept in mind.

3. Reducing agents—Vasoconstrictors used in anesthetic solution are unstable. They might get oxidized and discoloration of the solution occurs. To prevent this, small quantity of sodium metabisulphite is added to the anesthetic solution. Sodium metabisulphite has greater affinity to oxygen compared to the vasoconstrictors and thus prevents its oxidation. Sulphites may result in allergic reactions. In some anesthetic preparations capryl hydro-cuprinotoxin is added as a preservative as this does not cause any allergic reactions.

4. Preservative—Preservatives are added to anesthetic solution to maintain the sterility and to increase their shelf life. Usually methyl or propyl paraben is used as preservative. Parabens are known to cause allergic reactions.

5. Antifungal agents—A small quantity of thymol is added to anesthetic solution to prevent any fungal growth.

6. Vehicle—Ringer's solution is used to dissolve all the above constituents and render the anesthetic solution compatible with tissue fluids.

2 Nervous System

STRUCTURE OF NERVOUS SYSTEM

The nervous system comprises of neurons which are specialized tissues, with the ability to co-relate, integrate and rapidly conduct sensations such as touch, pain and temperature to the nerve centers and carry the responses back to the viseral and other organs of the body. A neuron is made up of a cell body, which gives out number of processes called dendrites. Apart from these dendrites, a long process extends from the cell body called axon (Fig. 2-1). The axon can extend to various lengths through the body. Axon contains gelatinous axoplasm encased in a membrane, which separates it from extracellular fluid.

The vital difference between the dendrite and the axon is that, the impulses from the dendrites travel up to the cell body, whereas an axon transmits the impulses away from the cell body. The axon is covered by a rolled myelin sheath, which intercepts at regular intervals. Between two segments of myelin sheaths, the axon membrane is exposed to tissue fluid. The area of interceptions are called as nodes of Ranvier. The myelin layer is covered by a layer of cytoplasm called neurilemma, which encloses a Schwann cell at the outer part (Fig. 2-2). This Schwann cell is responsible for the formation of the myelin sheath. A connective tissue layer called endoneurium holds together a number of nerve fibers forming a bundle or fasciculi. Several such fasciculi are covered and held together by a dense layer of connective tissue called epineurium (Fig. 2-3). The size of the nerve fiber varies from thick to fine. The thick

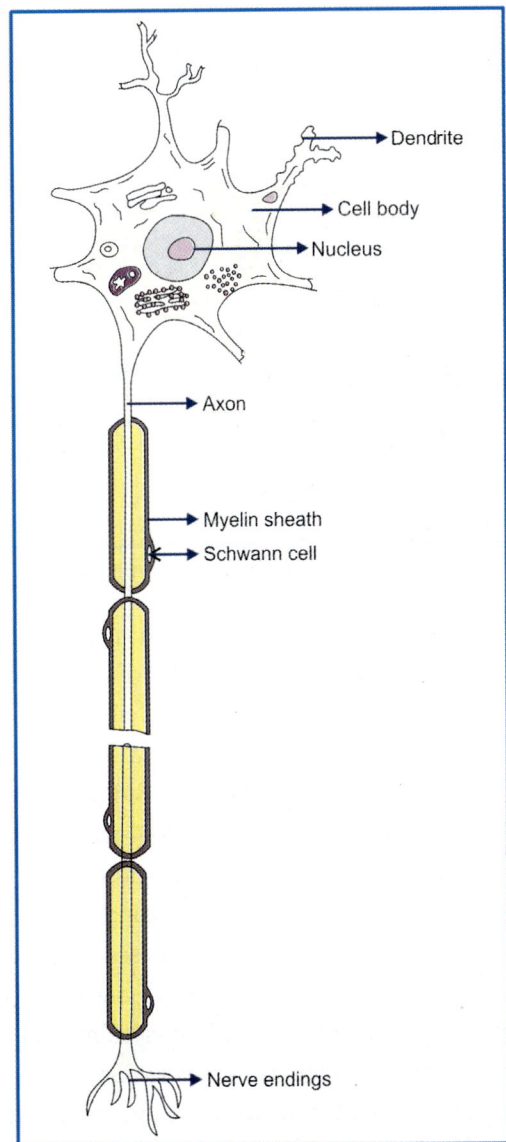

Fig. 2-1: Diagram of a multipolar neuron

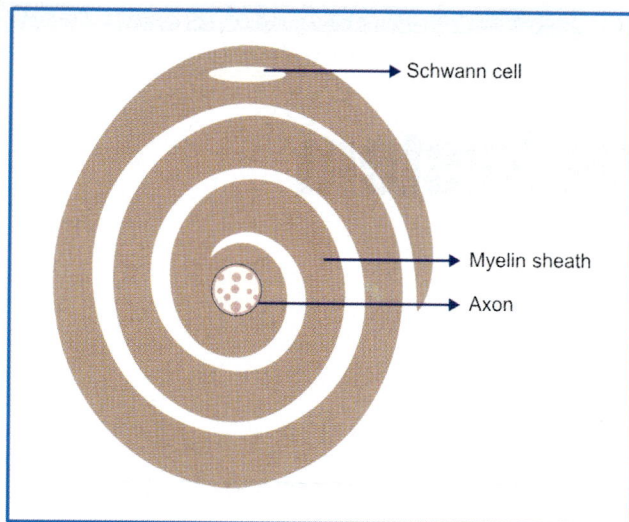

Fig. 2-2: Cross section of a myelinated nerve fiber

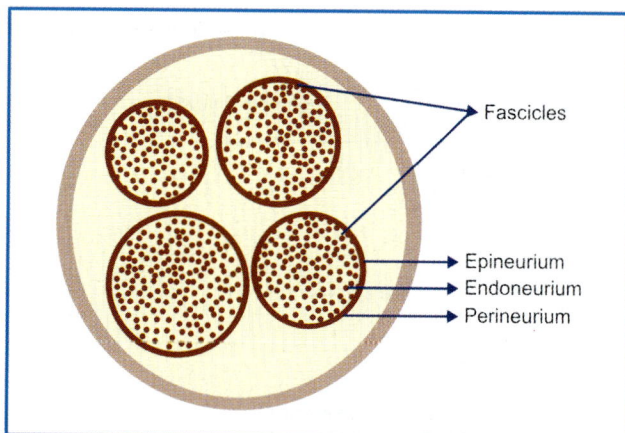

Fig. 2-3: Cross section of a nerve bundle

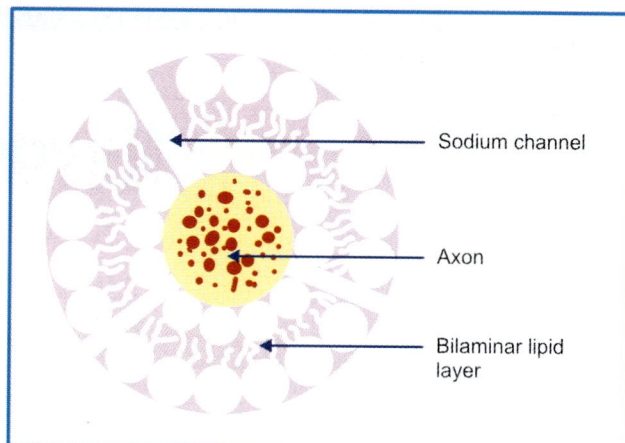

Fig. 2-4: Diagrammatic representation of cross section of a neuron

head faces outwards and the hydrophobic ends faces inwards (Fig. 2-4). Proteins are embedded in the lipid matrix. Ion channels lined by protein globules traverse the membrane. These channels are dynamically active and open and close influenced by external electrical or chemical forces.

PATHWAY OF PAIN SENSATION

Sensations of pain, touch, pressure and temperature from the facial region are carried from the peripheral nerves to the semi-lunar ganglion of the trigeminal nerve (Fig. 2-5). The central fibers from the ganglion enter the pons and 50% of these fibers divide into: a) ascending, and b) descending fibers. The rest of the 50% along with ascending fibers terminate in the main sensory nucleus. The descending fibers terminate in the spinal tract nucleus. The ascending fibers carry sensations of tactile sensibility and the descending fibers carry the sensation of pain and temperature. The proprioceptive sensation from the muscles of mastication and facial muscles are carried by the motor nerve of the trigeminal nerve, pass through motor nucleus and terminate in mesencephalic nucleus. The ascending fibers from the spinal tract nucleus join the other sensory fibers in the mesencephalic nucleus, cross the median plane, ascend and terminate in the postventral nucleus of thalamus. The fibers from the thalamus are carried to the cerebral cortex.

nerve fibers are myelinated and thinner fibers are unmyelinated. Based on the diameter of the nerve fibre they can be classified as A, B, and C. 'A' fibers are further classified as alpha (α)- 15-20 μm, beta (β) – 8-15 μm, gamma (γ) – 4-8 μm, and delta (δ)- 3-4 μm, A and B are myelinated fibers. C fibers (0.5 to 4 μ) are thin and unmyelinated. Type 'A' fibers supply muscles, spindles, and tendons. Type 'B' fibers are preganglionic afferent or efferent fibers which transmit impulses from viscera, skin and mucous membrane. Type 'C' are fibers in the postganglionic autonomic nervous system and carry sensation of pain, touch and temperature.

The nerve membrane which plays an important role in impulse transmission is made up of double layered phospholipid molecules. The hydrophilic

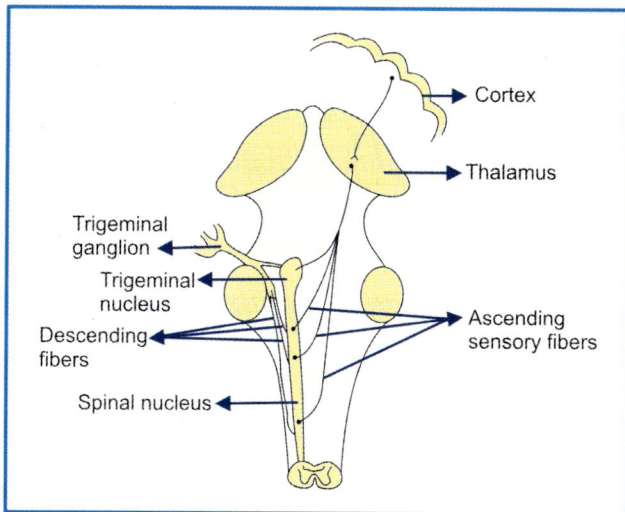

Fig. 2-5: Pain pathway

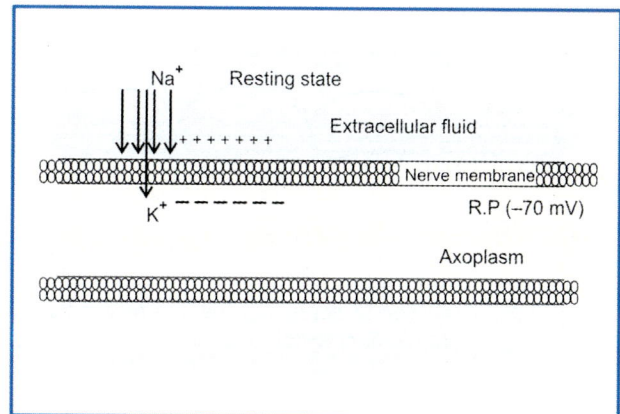

Fig. 2-6: Diagrammatic representation of resting state of a nerve

PHYSIOLOGY OF NERVE IMPULSE CONDUCTION

Propogation of a nerve impulse in response to a stimulus occurs by a complex physiologic activity, which can be explained thus: In a resting nerve there is low sodium ion concentration and a higher potassium concentration. Outside the nerve membrane, the tissue fluid concentration of Na^+ ions is higher. This creates a concentration gradient of electrolytes across the membrane which is usually around – 70 mV. Apart from this, there is low concentration of Cl^+ and Ca^{++} ions within the neural tissue. There is a continuous passive exchange of ions across the membrane with a tendency for sodium ions to diffuse into the nerve. The diffused sodium ions are continuously being removed by sodium pump, which regulates the constant tissue gradient. This state in the nerve is termed as resting potential (Fig. 2-6).

When the nerve is stimulated by any of the causes the nerve membrane becomes momentarily highly permeable to Na^+ ions (Fig. 2-7) which brings down the tissue gradient from –70 mV to + 20 or + 40 mV. This reversal of Na^+ ion concentration initiates an action potential which transmits the nerve impulse along the nerve fibers. This process is called depolarization (Fig. 2-8).

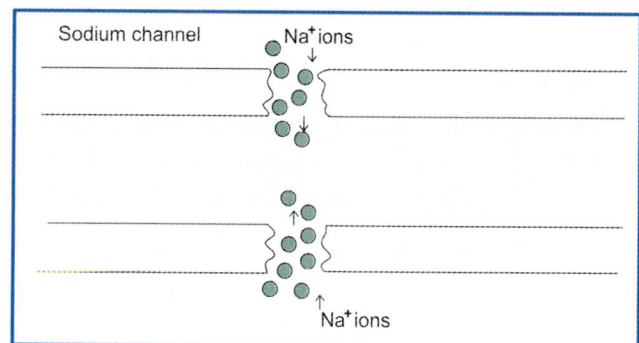

Fig. 2-7: Na^+ ions entering the nerve through the sodium chanel

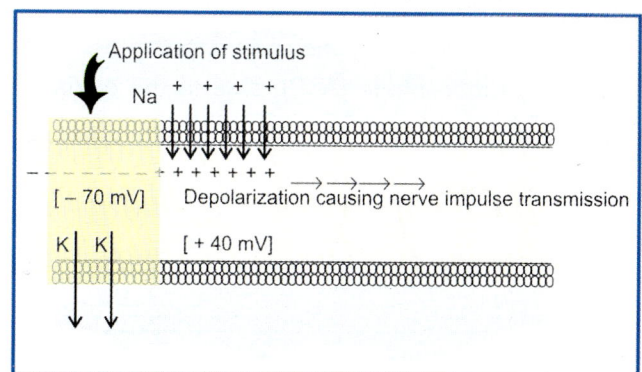

Fig. 2-8: Diagrammatic representation of depolarization

In a non-myelinated nerve fiber, the impulse travels along the nerve by segmental depolarization of adjacent nerve length while repolarization follows rapidly. This results in slow conduction of the nerve impulse. In a

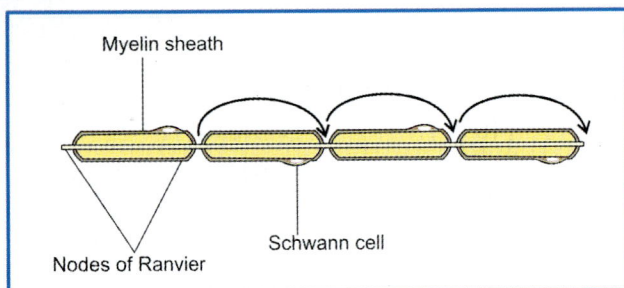

Fig. 2-9: Conduction of nerve impulse in a myelinated nerve fiber-saltatory effect

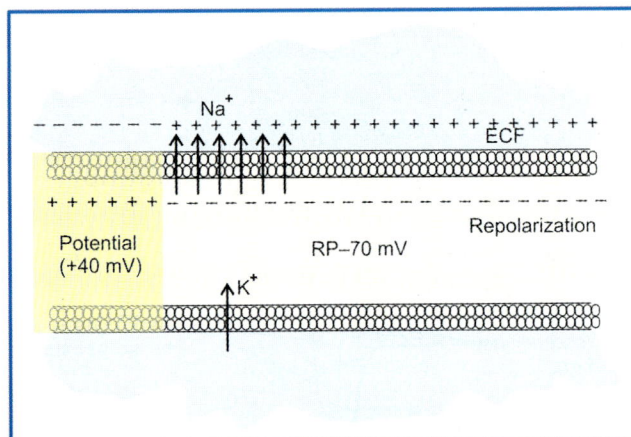

Fig. 2-11: Diagrammatic representation of repolarization

myelinated nerve fiber, the sodium diffusion is at the nodes of Ranvier. Hence the action potential hops from one node to the other which is termed as saltatory effect (Fig. 2-9). In saltatory action the ion current at each successive nodes becomes smaller until the firing threshold is reached. To effectively block the transmission of impulses in a myelinated nerve the anesthetic solution should at least bathe 2 or 3 successive nodes (Fig. 2-10). The conduction of impulse is faster in myelinated fibers. As the distance between two nodes of Ranvier increases the speed of conduction also increases.

After the influx of Na$^+$ ions during depolarization, potassium ions diffuse out of the nerve down the concentration gradient bringing back the potential to normal. This is termed as repolarization (Fig. 2-11). During repolarization, Na$^+$ ions present in excess within the nerve is removed by the sodium pump using the adenosine triphosphate (ATP). Due to the oxidative

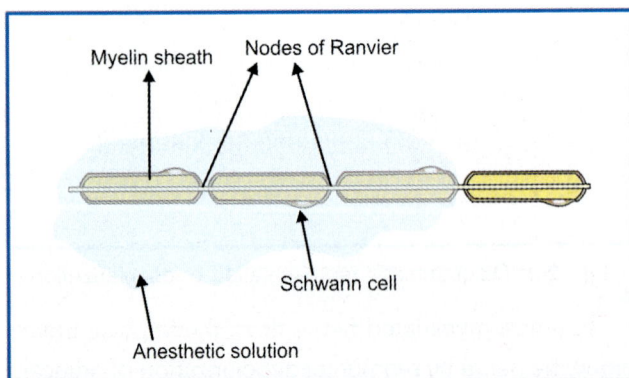

Fig. 2-10: Diagrammatic representation of anesthetic solution covering three consecutive nodes of Ranvier

metabolism of ATP the necessary energy is created to activate the sodium pump. At the same time potassium ions enter back into the nerve. The nerve returns to the resting potential of –70 mV.

MODE OF ACTION

A number of theories have been put forward to explain the mechanism of action of anesthetic drugs on the nerve membrane.

Humoral Theory

It is postulated that acetylcholine is responsible for the transmission of the impulse conduction. The lack of any definitive evidence of a chemical action and since there is dissimilarity between acteylcholine and local anesthetics. This is not an acceptable theory.

Calcium Displacement Theory

Role of calcium in nerve block is still being disputed. However it is beyond doubt that it does cause certain amount of nerve membrane excitability. The theory postulates that the local anesthetic molecules displace the calcium from their receptor sites and in turn get attached to them. This binding of the anesthetic molecules to the receptor sites is supposed to prevent sodium ion influx into the nerve.

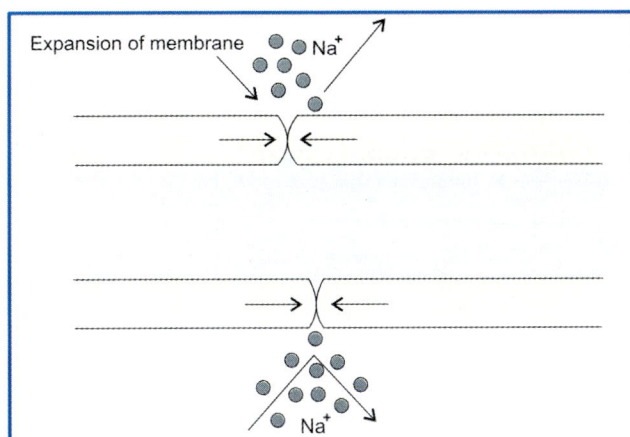

Fig. 2-12: Diagrammatic representation of expansion of membrane resulting in closure of sodium channel thereby preventing Na+ ion entry into the nerve

Membrane Expansion Theory

According to this theory as the anesthetic solution penetrates the nerve it diffuses through the membrane. This results in expansion of the membrane, which leads to the closure of specific channels through which the Na^+ ions diffuse into the nerve (Fig. 2-12).

Specific Receptor Theory

This has been the most favored theory, which postulates that the anesthetic molecule binds with specific protein receptor in the sodium channel which in turn blocks the diffusion of the sodium ions into the axoplasm. Local anesthetic cations infiltrates to the specific receptor-binding site through the lipophilic transmembrane route. Once the protein binding occurs it blocks the entry of Na^+ ions and thereby blocks conduction.

MODULATION OF PAIN

Gate Control Theory

In 1965 Melzack and Wall explained the Gate control theory, which explains the method of modulation of pain sensation. Pain sensation carried by 'C' fibers are slow in transmission compared to the thicker A-delta fibers. The tactile sensation conducted by thicker fibers can alter the transmission of pain sensation, thus facilitating or preventing its onward transmission. This process can occur either in spinal nucleus or in caudal nucleus of the trigeminal nerve.

Pain suppression (analgesia) system in the brain and spinal cord : Descending control system from the cortical centers are also likely to influence the process of facilitation or inhibition of pain transmission. The degree to which a person reacts to pain varies tremendously. This may be the result from capability of the brain itself to suppress transmission of pain signals by activating a pain control system called analgesic system. Stimulation of the areas in the periaquadctal gray and raphe magnus can stimulate neurotransmitters (encephalins and seratonin) to block the signals of pain being transmitted at the dorsal spinal roots (Fig. 2-13). The neurotransmitters cause both presynaptic and postsynaptic inhibition of pain coming through type 'C' and type 'A' (delta) fibers at the dorsal horn. This is effected by prevention of release of substance 'P' at substantia gelatinosa of the dorsal horn (Figs 2-14A and B).

Limbic system, the site of emotion when stimulated can initiate the pain inhibitory system. This is influenced by psychological fear, previous experience and the threshold of tolerance of pain. A person with higher tolerance and mind set cannot feel the pain for which a

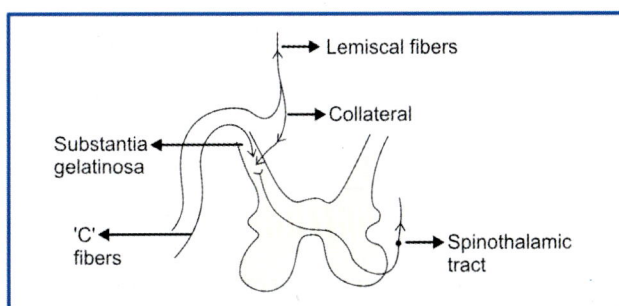

Fig. 2-13: Gate control at the dorsal horn. Lemiscal fibers through collateral branch prevents substance 'P' being liberated

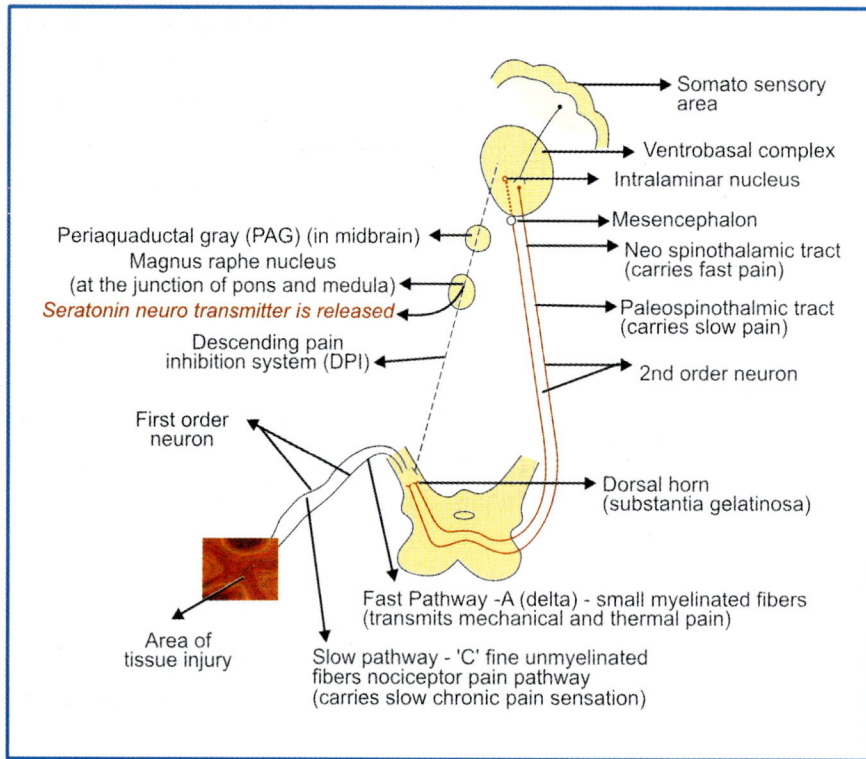

Fig. 2-14A: Diagrammatic representation of descending pain inhibition system. Opioid peptide encephalin related at the dorsal horn by the descending pain inhibition system combines with receptors of afferent pain carrying neuron at the dorsal horn and prevents the release of substance 'P' the neurotransmitter. Thus, the further conduction of pain is inhibited

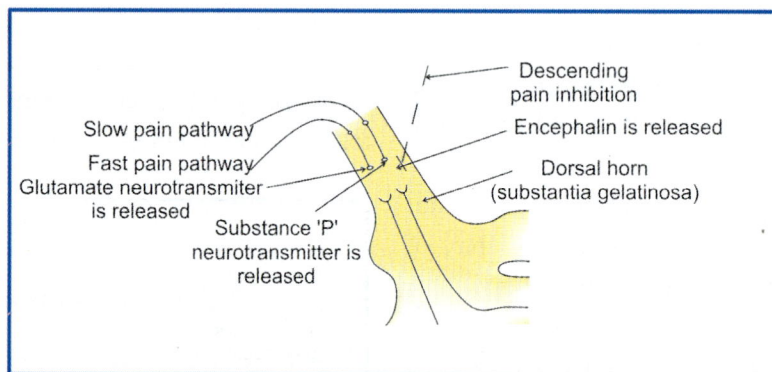

Fig. 2-14B: Detailed view of the dorsal horn

person with lower tolerance level might react intensively. The tolerance level might vary from time to time in an individual. In the author's own experience, a patient had all her teeth removed without any type of anesthesia. This type of high threshold to pain must have been influenced by the descending control system.

3

Trigeminal Nerve

Trigeminal nerve is the 5th cranial nerve (Fig. 3-1), consisting of a large sensory root and a smaller motor root. The sensory root arises from the pons with the motor root on the medial aspect. The sensory root reaches the gasserian ganglion situated in the Meckel's cave of the petrous bone. From the ganglion, the three branches of the trigeminal nerve namely ophthalmic, maxillary and mandibular are given out. The ophthalmic division passes through the superior orbital fissure and gives out the lacrimal, frontal and nasocilliary branches. The maxillary nerve leaves the skull through foramen rotundum to supply the maxillary area. The mandibular nerve emerges through foramen ovale to supply the mandibular region. The motor root of the trigeminal nerve passes below the trigeminal ganglion, through the foramen ovale and joins the mandibular nerve.

OPHTHALMIC NERVE

Ophthalmic nerve is the 1st division of the trigeminal

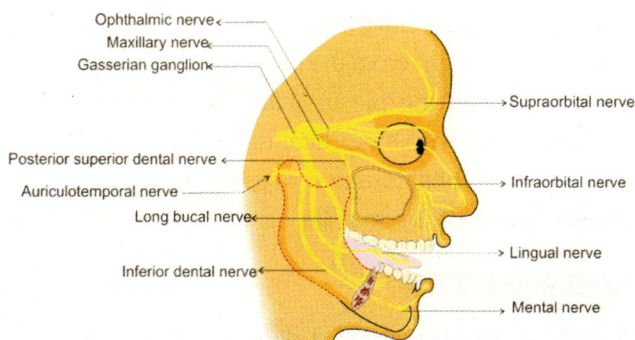

Fig. 3-1: Trigeminal nerve and its important branches

nerve. It is purely a sensory nerve and is the shortest of the three branches of the trigeminal nerve. It enters the orbit through the superior orbital fissure and supplies the eye ball, conjunctiva, paranasal sinuses, lacrimal glands and skin over nose, eyelids and forehead. Its main branches are nasociliary, frontal and lacrimal nerve.

MAXILLARY NERVE

This is the second division of the trigeminal nerve and is entirely sensory. After emerging from the foramen rotundum, it lies in the pterygopalatine fossa and gives out branches to the sphenopalatine ganglion. The posterior superior alveolar nerve branches out in the pterygopalatine fossa (Fig. 3-2), runs on the posterior surface of the maxilla and enters the maxillary sinus. Before entering the maxillary sinus, it gives out branches which supply the gingival region. In the maxillary sinus the nerve forms a plexus and supplies the molar teeth.

Sphenopalatine Ganglion

Branches from the maxillary nerve pass through the sphenopalatine ganglion without any functional relationship with the ganglion. From the ganglion the following branches are given out.

Greater and Lesser Palatine Nerves

The greater palatine nerve enters the palate through the greater palatine foramen and supplies the mucous

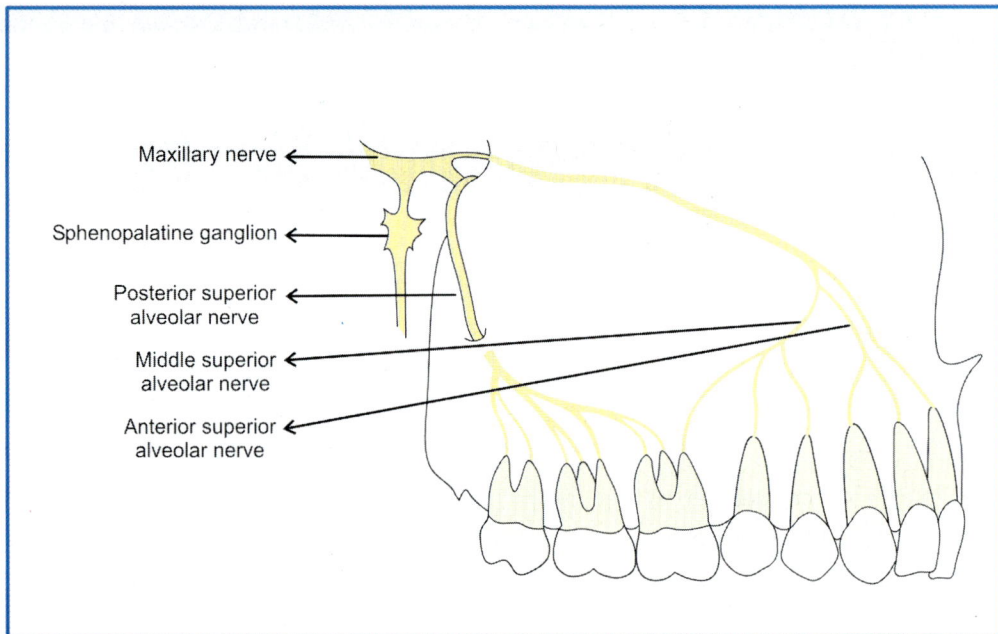

Fig. 3-2: Maxillary nerve and its main branches

membrane of the palate and gingiva from the molar teeth up to canine region. Occasionally, branches from this nerve, may supply the palatal roots of the molar teeth. The lesser palatine nerve passes through the lesser palatine foramina and supplies the mucous membrane of the soft palate, uvula and tonsils.

Posterior Nasal Branches

These branches supply the posterior region of nasal cavity including the inferior nasal concha and middle meatus.

Orbital Branches

Few branches supply the periosteum of the orbit.

Zygomatic Branch

It enters through the superior orbital fissure, passes over the lateral wall of the orbit and supplies the skin over the cheek and temporal region through zygomaticofacial and zygomaticotemporal branches.

Long Sphenopalatine Branch

This nerve is also called as nasopalatine nerve which runs along the septum of the nose and enters the palate through the incisive canal and incisive foramen. It supplies the mucous membrane of anterior region of palate and gingiva from canine to canine teeth region.

The maxillary nerve, after the division of the superior alveolar nerve, enters the infraorbital groove through the infraorbital canal to emerge through the infraorbital foramen. During its passage through the infraorbital groove, the maxillary nerve gives out the middle superior alveolar nerve. This nerve forms a plexus and supplies the pre-molar teeth apart from supplying the mesiobuccal root of the first molar tooth. In the infraorbital canal the anteriosuperior alveolar nerve emerges and passes through a bony canal and forms a plexus over the incisor and canine teeth. Branches from the plexus supply these teeth. There is a possibility that fibers from the other side of the midline might cross over to form the plexus. A few fibers might join the plexus with the middle superior alveolar nerve. The infraorbital nerve after coming out from the infraorbital foramen supplies the skin over the anterior region of the maxilla.

MANDIBULAR NERVE

Mandibular nerve is the 3rd division of the trigeminal nerve and is a mixed nerve. Immediately after emerging

Table 3.1: Maxillary nerve – 2nd division of maxillary nerve

Place of division	Branches	Area of supply
In the cranium	Meningeal branch	Supplies dura mater in the middle cranial fossa
In the pterygoid fossa	1. Branch to the sphenopalatine ganglion Ganglionic branches	
	a. Greater palatine nerve	• Innervates mucous membrane of the hard palate and the gingiva on the palatal aspect upto pre-molar teeth region.
	b. Lesser palatine nerve	• Innervates mucous membrane of soft palate, uvula and tonsils.
	c. Posterior nasal branches	• Innervates mucous membrane covering the posterior part of nasal cavity.
	d. Orbital branches	• Innervates periosteum of orbit, sphenoid and ethmoid air sinuses.
	e. Zygomatic branch	• Skin covering the zygomatic bone is supplied by zygomatico facial while the skin over temporal region supplied by zygomatico temporal branch.
	f. Nasopalatine nerve	• Innervates mucous membrane of nasal septum, anterior region of palate and gingiva.
	2. Posteriosuperior alveolar nerve	• Innervates maxillary molars, mucous membrane in the buccal region in that area including gingiva.
In the infraorbital groove	Middle superioalveolar nerve	• Innervates pre-molar teeth, mucous membrane of the buccal region including gingiva and mucous membrane of maxillary sinus.
In the infraorbital canal Emerges from the infraorbital foramen.	Anteriosuperior alveolar nerve	• Innervates maxillary anterior teeth and mucous membrane of anterior region of nasal cavity.
	1. Infraorbital nerve	
	a. Nasal branches	Skin over the nose
	b. Superior labial branches	Skin and mucous membrane of the anterior region cheek and lip.

from the foramen ovale, the mandibular nerve gives out a meningeal branch and also a nerve to the medial pterygoid muscle. The main nerve then divides into posterior and anterior trunks (Fig. 3-3).

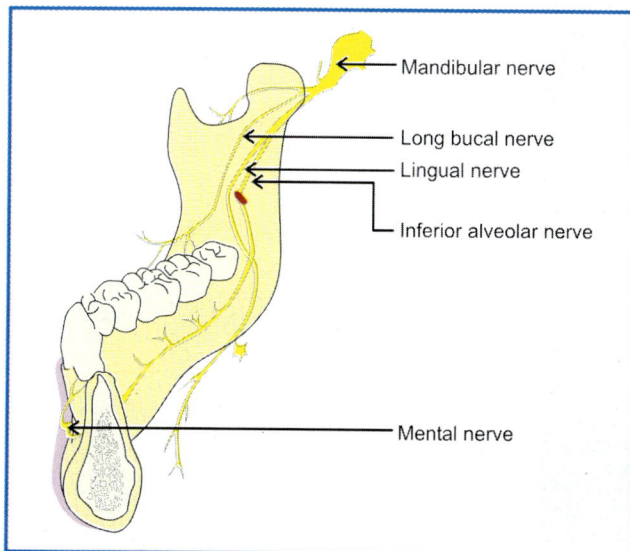

Fig. 3-3: Mandibular nerve and its branches

Meningeal branch enters the middle cranial fossa through foramen spinosum and supplies the dura mater. The medial pterygoid muscle branch supplies that particular muscle. The medial pterygoid nerve also gives out few fibers which pass through otic ganglion and innervate the two tensor muscles.

The anterior smaller trunk of the mandibular nerve further divides into buccal, massetric, temporal and lateral pterygoid branches. Except the buccal, rest of the nerve branches are motor nerves supplying the respective muscles.

Buccal nerve branch passes between 2 heads of lateral pterygoid muscle, crosses the ramus of mandible on to the buccinator muscle to supply the mucous membrane and skin over the buccinator muscle area. It also supplies the gingiva in the molar region. The course of the nerve across the anterior border of the ramus varies, sometimes being at a higher level and sometimes at a lower level.

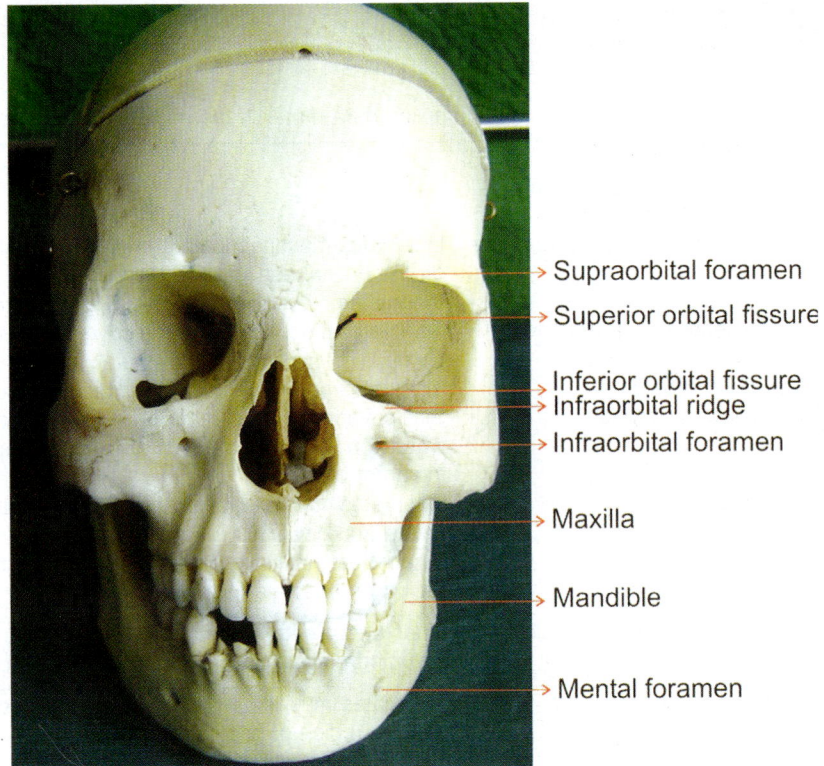

Fig. 3-4: Frontal view of skull showing various foramina

- Supraorbital foramen
- Superior orbital fissure
- Inferior orbital fissure
- Infraorbital ridge
- Infraorbital foramen
- Maxilla
- Mandible
- Mental foramen

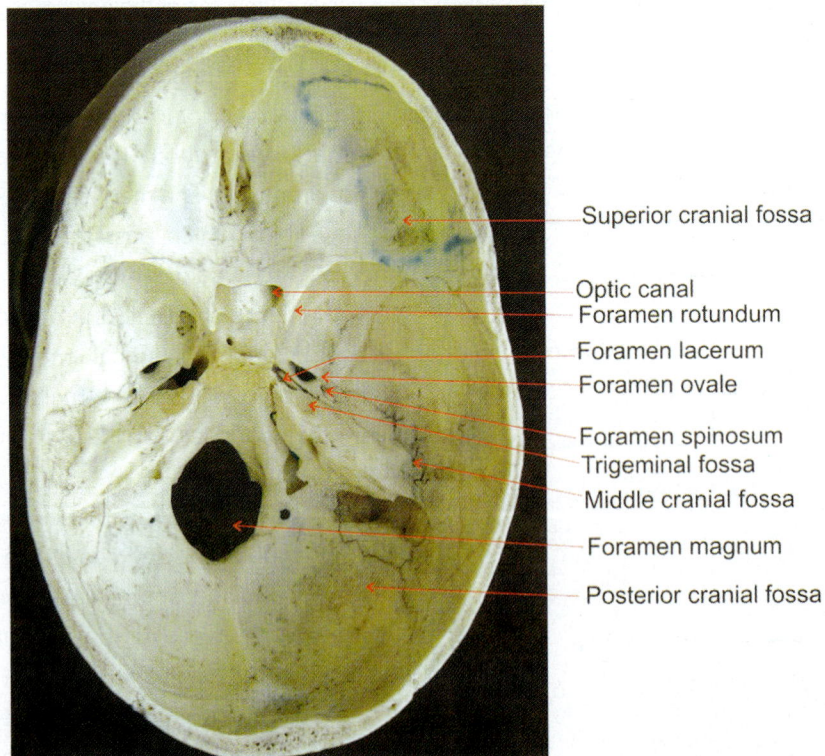

Fig. 3-5: Internal surface of the base of skull showing the foramina through which branches of trigeminal nerve enter from the skull

- Superior cranial fossa
- Optic canal
- Foramen rotundum
- Foramen lacerum
- Foramen ovale
- Foramen spinosum
- Trigeminal fossa
- Middle cranial fossa
- Foramen magnum
- Posterior cranial fossa

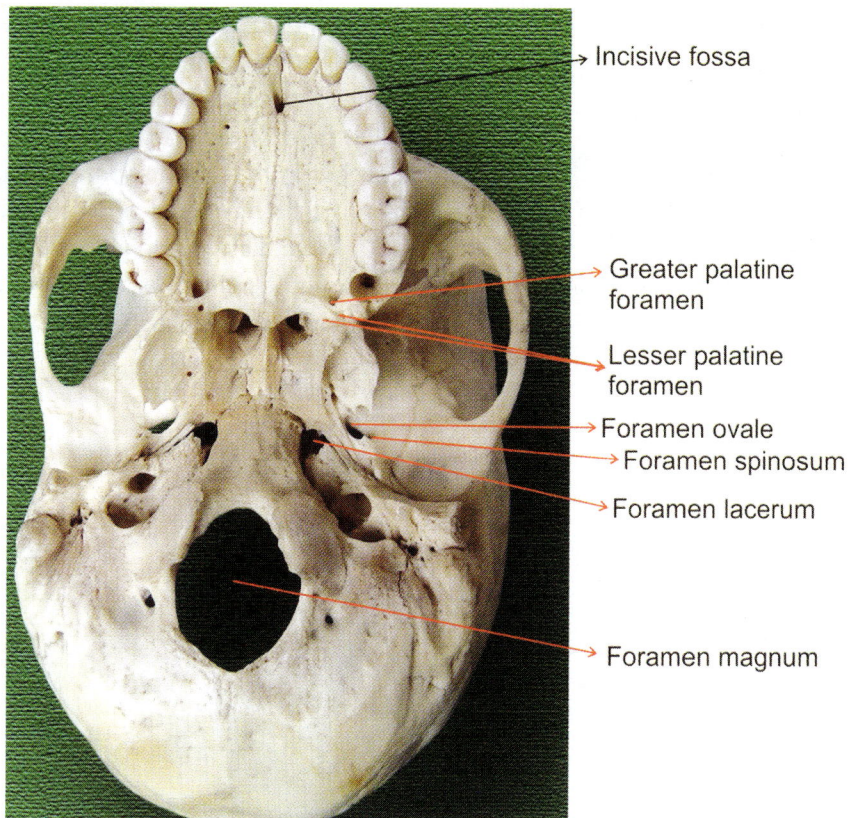

Fig. 3-6: External surface of the base of skull showing the foramina through which the trigeminal nerve branches leave the skull

The larger posterior trunk of mandibular nerve divides into auriculotemporal, inferior alveolar and lingual nerves, all of which are sensory.

The auriculotemporal arises by two roots, which encircles the middle meningeal artery, and passes behind the temporomandibular joint capsule. In this lateral course, it emerges close to the superior aspect of parotid gland. The nerve supplies skin over the temple, ear and external auditory meatus, tympanic membrane, parotid gland and temporomandibular joint. The fibers to the parotid gland carry the secretomotor fibers from the glossopharyngeal nerve through the otic ganglion.

The Inferior Alveolar Nerve

After branching from the main nerve, the inferior alveolar nerve passes below the lateral pterygoid muscle and runs between the ramus and sphenomandibular ligament. Before entering the mandibular foramen, it gives out a branch to the mylohyoid muscle and within the canal it gives out number of branches which innervate molar and premolar teeth. At the mental foramen area it branches into incisive and mental nerve branches. The incisive nerve supplies the canine and incisor teeth. The central incisors and sometimes the lateral incisors are supplied from nerve plexus from the opposite side. The mental nerve emerges from the mental foramen and supplies the mucous membrane and gingiva in the premolar incisor region. It also supplies the skin over the chin and lower lip. The inferior alveolar nerve is usually anesthetized at the mandibular foramen region. Sometimes patients might feel slight pain even after blocking of this nerve. This may be due to tiny branches of nerve arising from the inferior alveolar nerve at a higher level and inervating the last molar tooth.

Lingual Nerve

This nerve supplies anterior 2/3rd of the tongue, mucous membrane of the floor of the mouth and the gingiva on the lingual aspect. After branching out from the posterior trunk, it unites with the chorda tympani branch of the facial nerve. It passes below the attachment of the pterygomandibular raphe at which point it is closely placed to the medial surface of the mandible corresponding to the roots of the 3rd molar tooth. The lingual nerve continues between the hyoglossus and mylohyoid muscles and divides into terminal branches in the floor of the mouth. Few terminal branches join branches from the glossopharyngeal nerve at the tip of the tongue. The lingual nerve also gives out branches to the submandibular ganglion. The secretomotor fibers are carried by the chorda tympani nerve to the submandibular and sublingual glands.

4

Assessment and General Examination

Prior to administration of anesthetic injection it is mandatory to undertake a complete assessment of the patient regarding the general health. A detailed history should be recorded and the patient should be subjected to a general medical examination.

HISTORY

- Chief complaint
- History of present illness
- Past history
  - Dental
  - Medical
- Family history
- Personal habits
- Past treatment history
- Allergic reactions
- Medications
- Pregnancy

EXAMINATION

- General medical examination
- Cardiovascular
- Respiratory
- Head and neck
- Oral cavity

Specific questions should elicit presence of any systemic diseases relevant to dentistry

1. **A**llergies
2. **B**lood disorders
3. **C**ardiac and respiratory conditions
4. **D**iabetes – drugs taken
5. **E**xistence of low or high BP
6. **F**aints and epilepsy
7. **G**ynecological problems and pregnancy
8. **H**epatic and kidney ailments

If required, blood investigations or any other investigation should be undertaken. In case of medically compromised patients it is advisable to seek a physician's opinion as to the patient's fitness to undergo surgical procedures under local anesthesia.

Allergic Reactions

Patients many a time voluntarily disclose during history taking that they are allergic to certain drugs. The patient could be allergic to antibiotics, analgesics or even local anesthetic agents. In case the patient does not come out with voluntary disclosure, specific questions regarding allergies could be sought from the patient. It is necessary to enquire about previous injections for any dental treatment. The name of the drug or the anesthetic would be useful information. Patient might relate of previous fainting during dental treatment. This might be just syncope or it could be an allergic reaction. Details regarding such fainting should give a fairly good idea as to the cause. The local anesthetic drug used in this country is lignocaine. This amide group of anesthetic by itself does not cause any allergic reaction but one of the constituents of the anesthetic solution like the preservative on the antioxidant may be responsible for the allergic reaction. If further investigation does not reveal the real causative factor of the allergy, it may be wise to use plain anesthetic solution or subject the patient to allergic test. Allergic reaction to other drugs like analgesics and antibiotics should be borne in mind before prescribing drugs after dental treatment.

Bleeding Disorders

If the patient is afflicted with a bleeding disorder for a long time, the patient himself will usually disclose the same during the general history taking, since the family physician would have warned the patient the importance of voluntary disclosure. However, it is necessary to enquire about previous dental procedures especially extraction of teeth. Prolonged bleeding after extraction of teeth should be properly investigated. If there is a definite history of bleeding a complete blood investigation should be ordered. In patients with history of prolonged bleeding local anesthetic injection should be restricted to infiltration techniques.

Cardiac and Respiratory Condition

Patients with cardiac ailments usually present all the records along with previous investigations. This could give a definite picture as to whether the patient is suffering from valuvlar disease, cardiac infarction or arrhythmias. In patients with valvular ailments requiring dental surgical procedure, the standard preoperative antibiotic regime should be followed. While giving dental anesthesia extra care should be taken to properly disinfect the area of needle penetration. In cases of myocardial infarction, the patient's cardiac function would have reduced and he may find it difficult to cope with the stress induced by dental treatment. It is advisable to avoid any routine procedures for a period of 6 months. If it is an emergency treatment, the patient should be premedicated and the patient's physician should be consulted before proceeding with the dental treatment. In patients with anginal attacks it is advantageous to take the physicians

instructions regarding the regime of premedication before instituting any dental surgical procedure. Emergency drugs should be readily available in case of anginal attacks during procedure. In all cardiac ailments the important factor is councelling the patient before dental treatment. Assurance from the dental surgeons and careful premedication does go a long way in preventing any complication during dental procedures.

Respiratory problems such as bronchial asthma and any infections of the respiratory system should be properly investigated. In asthmatic patients preoperative use of bronchodilators would help in smooth handling of dental problems.

Diabetes

This is a metabolic disorder affecting glucose metabolism. In a chronic diabetic patient, there could be several other changes like arteriosclerosis and kidney affections. Diabetic patients are prone to cardiac ailments and kidney diseases. Although there is a general awareness of this condition patient tend to neglect regular follow-ups. Some elderly patients might accidentally come to know about the condition during random investigations. Adminis-tering local anesthesia for routine dental treatment may not result in any complications but when extraction of teeth or minor surgery is to be undertaken there is always chances of infection and delayed wound healing. Preoperative administration of antibiotics and careful aseptic procedures should be followed in patients with controlled diabetes. In uncontrolled diabetic patients, if the dental treatment is not an emergency, blood sugar level should be brought under control with proper medication before taking up dental treatment. In emergency, the procedure should be undertaken under adequate antibiotic coverage. Patients who are insulin dependant, should not be treated for any dental ailment with an empty stomach.

Hypertension

Majority of patients do not undergo routine medical examination. Many cases of hypertension are detected during investigation for some other illness. Local anesthesia is not contraindicated in mild hypertensive patients. Over the age of 40 it is wise to record the blood pressure of patients routinely. In some patients with hypertension, climbing stairs or slight exertion increases the blood pressure. Such patients do require a few minutes of rest before any dental procedure is undertaken. Fear and anxiety can also cause alteration in blood pressure levels. Premedication before dental treatment is recommended in such patients. In patients with postural hypertension a few minutes rest should be given every time the chair position is changed.

Fainting and Epileptic Attacks

Fainting in most of the cases is due to fear and apprehension. Preoperative councelling, if necessary administration of premedication, and positioning the patient in semireclining position would be sufficient to prevent any untoward effect. Epileptic attacks sometimes may be triggered by fear or pain during dental treatment. A detailed history of epileptic attacks and the treatment being taken by the patient is necessary before undertaking dental procedure under local anesthesia. Reassurance and a painless procedure should prevent any compli-cation in these patients.

Pregnancy

All routine dental procedures should be avoided during the 1st trimester of pregnancy. It is better to avoid all type of antibiotics and analgesics, however in case of dental infections drugs should be prescribed in consultation with the attending gynecologist. Local anesthetics solution should be limited to minimum dosage. Position of dental chair should be made comfortable without reclining it further backwards.

Hospital Admissions

History regarding previous admissions, the nature of illness, any surgeries undertaken, and drugs administered will give a clear picture as to precautions to be taken during administration of local anesthesia.

Hepatic and Kidney Ailments

In cases of cirrhosis of liver and kidney ailments caution should be exercised while administring anesthetic drugs. Physicians opinion should be sought regarding further administration of drugs after dental treatment. Minimum dosage of anesthetic drug should be used to avoid toxic complications due to overdosage.

Methods of Local Anesthesia

Local anesthesia in dentistry is extensively used for various procedures. Different methods of local anesthesia are employed to suit each procedure. Basically local anesthesia in oral cavity can be achieved by two methods:

1. By application of local anesthetic agent on the surface of mucous membrane (Figs 5.1A and B).
2. By injecting the anesthetic solution into the tissues (Figs 5.2A and B).

BY APPLICATION OF LOCAL ANESTHETIC AGENT ON THE SURFACE OF MUCOUS MEMBRANE

By applying local anesthetic agent on the surface of mucous membrane, surface anesthesia is achieved within 5 minutes. For local application, the agents are dispensed in various forms for different applications:

a. Mouth rinses
b. Lozenges
c. Viscous liquid
d. Ointments and jelly
e. Topical solution
f. Aerosol spray
g. Use of ethyl chloride

Mouth Rinses

Mouth rinses containing anesthetic agent are useful when anesthesia of large areas of mucous membrane is desired. Here the patient swishes 5 to 10 ml of the solution for 1 or 2 minutes and discards it. This is useful in preventing

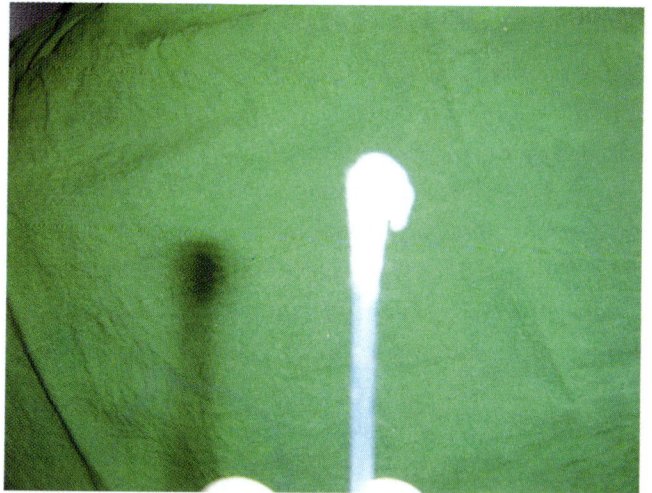

Fig. 5-1A: Anesthetic ointment carried on a cotton bud

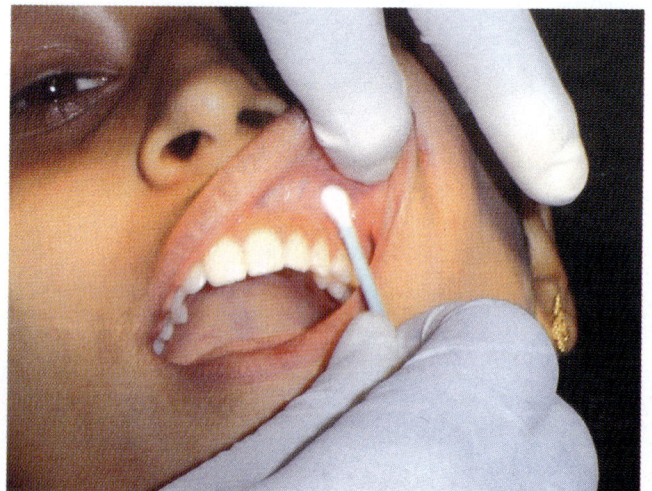

Fig. 5-1B: Application of local anesthetic agents (ointment) on the mucous membrane

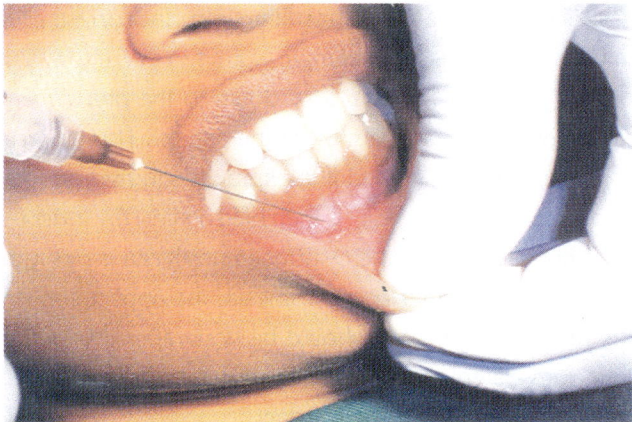

Fig. 5-2A: Injection of local anesthetic agent into the tissues

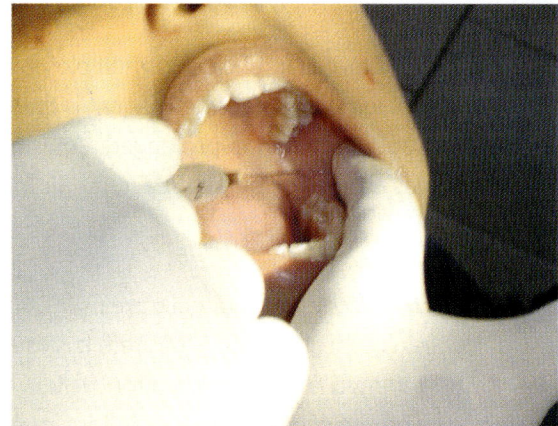

Fig. 5-2B: Injection of local anesthetic agent deep into tissues near to a nerve trunk

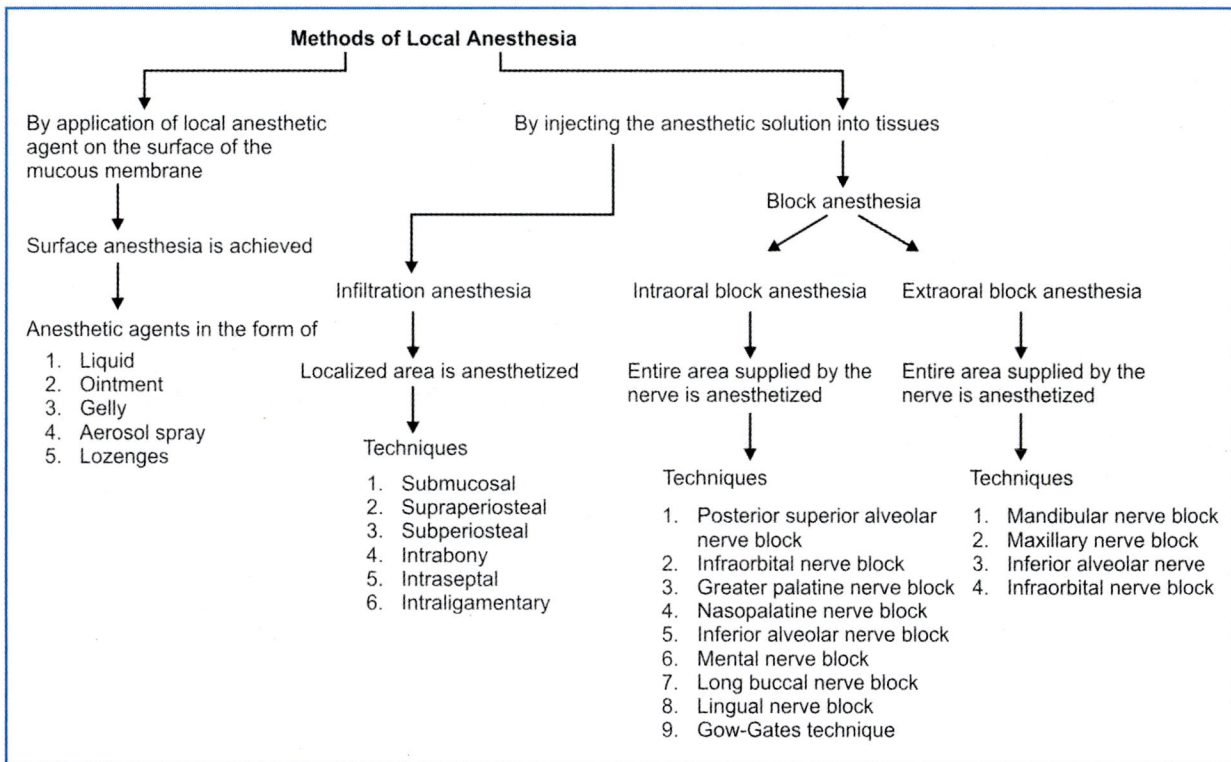

Methods of Local Anesthesia

By application of local anesthetic agent on the surface of the mucous membrane

Surface anesthesia is achieved

Anesthetic agents in the form of

1. Liquid
2. Ointment
3. Gelly
4. Aerosol spray
5. Lozenges

By injecting the anesthetic solution into tissues

Infiltration anesthesia

Localized area is anesthetized

Techniques

1. Submucosal
2. Supraperiosteal
3. Subperiosteal
4. Intrabony
5. Intraseptal
6. Intraligamentary

Block anesthesia

Intraoral block anesthesia

Entire area supplied by the nerve is anesthetized

Techniques

1. Posterior superior alveolar nerve block
2. Infraorbital nerve block
3. Greater palatine nerve block
4. Nasopalatine nerve block
5. Inferior alveolar nerve block
6. Mental nerve block
7. Long buccal nerve block
8. Lingual nerve block
9. Gow-Gates technique

Extraoral block anesthesia

Entire area supplied by the nerve is anesthetized

Techniques

1. Mandibular nerve block
2. Maxillary nerve block
3. Inferior alveolar nerve
4. Infraorbital nerve block

gaging during upper jaw impression, in patients who are sensitive to touch in the palatal region. This is also used in patients with multiple mouth ulcers or lichen planus. By anesthetizing the surface of mucous membrane the patients would be able to chew their food without much pain or burning sensation. The effect of superficial anesthesia usually lasts for about 15 to 30 minutes.

However the patient should be warned about accidental biting of the cheek or tongue during chewing. This generalized anesthetic effect in the oral cavity will certainly be uncomfortable to the patient but as the duration of the anesthetic effect is short and the patient is able to consume food without much pain, patients willingly tolerate this discomfort.

Lozenges

Anesthetic lozenges are used in case of multiple painful ulcers. The advantage of this anesthetic agent is that it is released slowly and its action is prolonged. Anesthetic agents in lozenges are not being manufactured in India.

Viscous Liquid

Anesthetic agent in viscous form or gelly are useful when surface anesthesia in specific areas is desired. It is usually applied to the required area with a cotton pellet. This application can be effectively used just before making intraoral injection, to reduce the pain during insertion of the needle. In case of solitary ulcers or lichen planus, the viscous solution and gelly can be applied to these areas to obtain surface anesthesia. The viscous solution can also be applied to the gingival region before undertaking prophylaxis of teeth. Viscous liquid and gelly is also used to smear over endotracheal tubes, before its placement. It can also be used in endoscopy for lubrication.

Ointments and Jelly

These two preparations have a similar useful purpose as that of viscous liquid. In dentistry the anesthetic agent in ointment form is more useful, since it can be applied to the required area without any chances of the agent spreading to surrounding areas as in the case of viscous liquid and jelly.

Xylocaine Topical Solution

This is available in 4% solution and has similar use as ointment. Surface anesthesia occurs within 2 to 5 minutes and persists upto 15-30 minutes. Its disadvantage is as in case of viscous and gelly, the liquid can flow down to other areas where anesthesia is not desired. The active agent in Xylocaine topical solution is lignocaine hydrochloride.

Aerosol Sprays

Aerosol sprays in the oral cavity provides surface anesthesia within few seconds. The disadvantage in this case is that it tends to flow, resulting in surface anesthesia in undesired areas. For example, sprays in the retromolar or soft palatal region can flow down to the pharyngeal region resulting in discomfort to the patient. This undesired effect can be avoided if the spray is squirted on to a cotton pellet and the pellet is then held against the mucous membrane in areas where surface anesthesia is desired.

In all types of surface anesthesia, the application on the mucous membrane should be done after drying the area with a sterile gauge as the presence of saliva dilutes the action of the anesthetic agent.

Use of Ethyl Chloride

Ethyl chloride when sprayed on skin or mucous membrane causes temporary numbness. This acts by refrigeration of the surface tissue. This can be effectively used to remove loose teeth or to nick an intraoral or extraoral abscess. On the skin ethyl chloride has to be sprayed till there is frost formation. While spraying extraorally one should cover the eyes properly. The numbness lasts only for few seconds.

LOCAL ANESTHESIA BY DEPOSITING THE ANESTHETIC SOLUTION IN THE TISSUES

The area anesthetized by this method depends upon the place of deposition of the anesthetic solution. This can be conveniently grouped under:
a. Infiltration anesthesia.
b. Nerve block anesthesia.

When anesthetic solution is superficially injected into the mucous membrane it diffuses in all directions. The terminal nerve endings in that area get anesthetized resulting in anesthesia of the local area. This is termed as infiltration anesthesia. When the solution is deposited in the deeper area near to a main nerve trunk, anesthesia is achieved in the entire region supplied by the nerve and its branches. This is termed as nerve block anesthesia. In case it is a mixed nerve the motor branch also gets anesthetized. Some authors have further sub-classified the nerve block into field block and nerve block anesthesia. The field block is achieved when main branch of a nerve is anesthetized. Nerve block anesthesia as mentioned earlier is achieved when a main trunk of the nerve is anesthetized. In this book the field block and nerve block have been grouped under a single group of nerve block anesthesia.

Infiltration Anesthesia

This is the most common type of anesthesia used for many of the minor oral surgical procedures undertaken in the oral cavity. Majority of extractions are done under infiltration anesthesia. This is a very safe method without any complications. The needle penetration into the tissues here is very minimal and hence there are no chances of accidental intravascular injections or injury to the nerve tissue.

There are many methods of infiltration which can be adopted depending upon the procedure.

1. Submucosal injection
2. Supraperiosteal injection
3. Subperiosteal injection
4. Intrabony injection
5. Intraseptal injection
6. Intraligamentary injection

Submucosal Injection (Fig. 5-3)

In this method the local anesthetic solution is deposited into the mucosal tissues to obtain anesthesia in that local area. The solution so deposited infiltrates in all directions anesthetizing the terminal nerve endings in that region. This can be used for undertaking minor oral surgical procedures in the lip or cheek region.

Supraperiosteal Injection (Figs 5.4A and B)

This is the most common method employed for many minor oral surgical procedures especially for extraction of teeth. The anesthetic solution in this method is deposited close to or on the surface of the periosteum (Fig. 5-4A). The solution diffuses through the periosteum and porous bone underneath to the periapical region of teeth. In this process, it anesthetizes the mucous membrane, periosteum, alveolar bone and the tooth. If

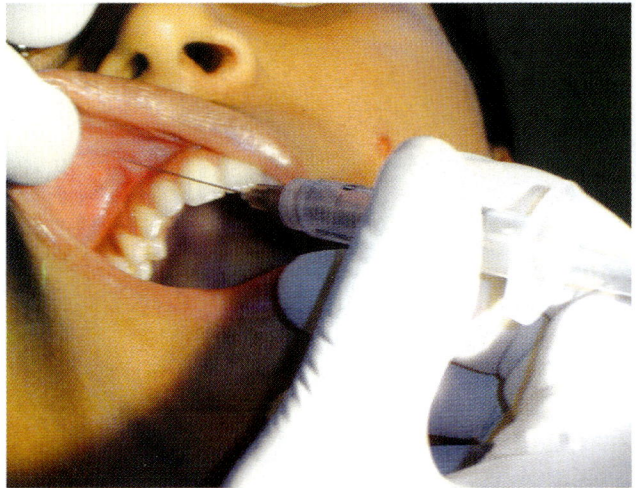

Fig. 5-3: Submucosal injection

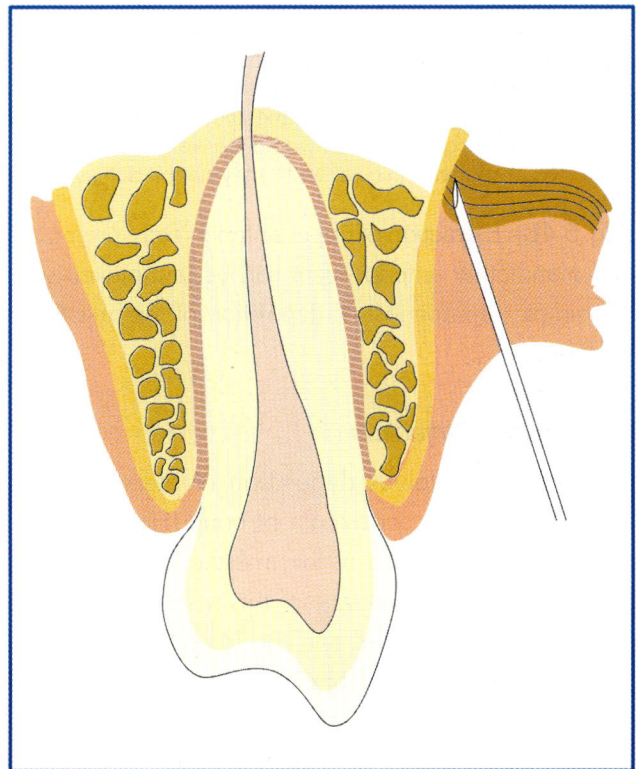

Fig. 5-4A: Diagrammatic representation of supraperiosteal injection

the injection is made away from the periosteal surface, the amount of anesthetic solution available to penetrate through periosteum and bone will be reduced. This results in ineffective anesthesia of that particular tooth

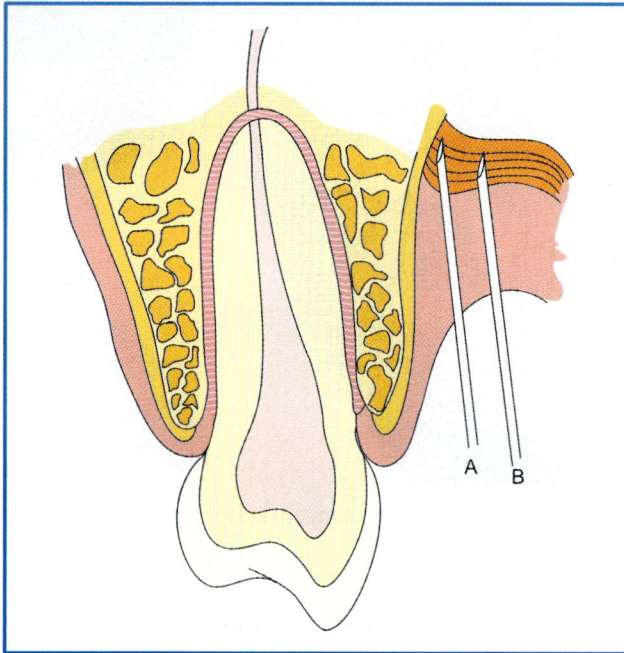

Fig. 5-4B: Diagrammatic representation of correct position of the needle (A). In 'B' position the needle tip is away from the bone. In this case the amount of anesthetic solution available for penetration of the bone would be very less. Hence, (anesthesia) of that particular tooth may not be achieved

(Fig. 5-4B). Extraction of upper anterior teeth, premolars and mandibular anterior teeth can be undertaken with this simple supraperiosteal deposition of the anesthetic solution.

Subperiosteal Injection

This method involves deposition of the anesthetic solution below the periosteum of bone (Fig. 5-5). This ensures faster diffusion of the anesthetic solution into the bone. The disadvantage of this method is that the injection is quite painful and the forced deposition of solution between the bone and periosteum causes separation of periosteum from the bone, which may result in post injection pain. This injection is not being used, as supraperiosteal injection results in satisfactory anesthesia and it also does not cause any pain during deposition of the solution.

Intrabony Injections

In this method of infiltration anesthesia, the anesthetic solution is deposited directly into the cancelous bone

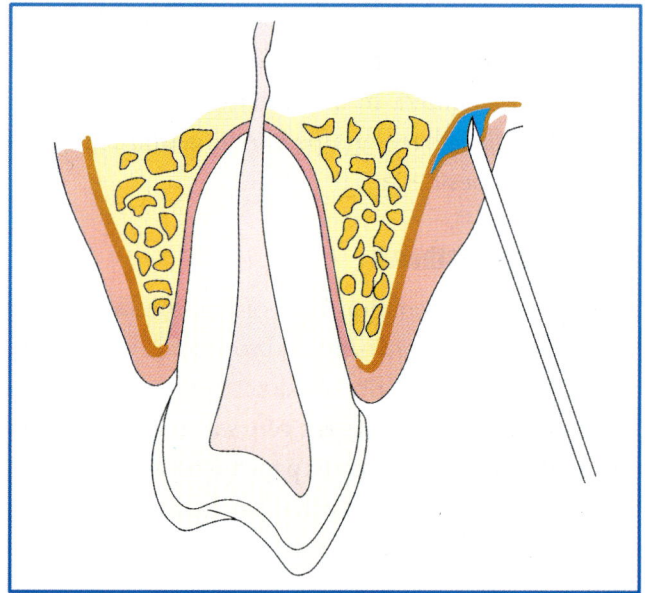

Fig. 5-5: Diagrammatic representation of subperiosteal deposition of anesthetic solution

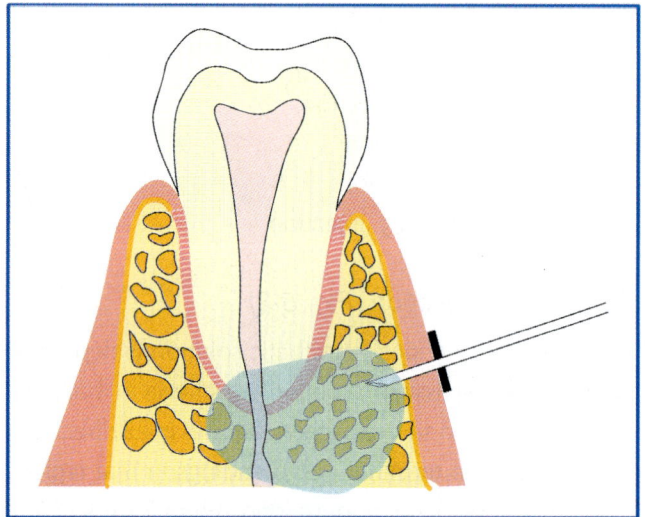

Fig. 5-6: Diagrammatic representation of Intrabony injection

close to the periapical region of the tooth (Fig. 5-6). For this purpose, first the surface of the mucous membrane at the region where the bur hole is to be made, is anesthetized by depositing a few drops of anesthetic solution in the submucosal region. A special bur is used to create a hole in the bone near the periapical region of the tooth. Through this opening the needle of the syringe is inserted and the anesthetic solution is deposited. To prevent back flow of the solution, a rubber stopper can be used on the needle. As this method involves drilling a hole in the bone to achieve local anesthesia, patient may not accept this method. This technique requires special type of burs and needle. With the presently available anesthetic agents supraperiosteal deposition is sufficient to obtain complete anesthesia of the area. In the present era of dental practice this elaborate technique of depositing the solution within the bone is not necessary.

Dentsply have introduced X-tip an intravenous anesthesia delivery system for deep pulpal anesthesia. This consists of a needle with guide sleeve which is attachable to a contra-angle handpiece. It is drilled directly into the cortex in between the roots of the teeth. The sleeve stays put like a button and can be used for subsequent injections. Anesthetic solution is injected into the bone through the sleeve. Anesthesia is supposed to be effective within a minute's time. The advantage of the method is that there is no anesthesia of the surrounding tissue and the patients feels very comfortable during and after the injection. This should be more useful in conservative and endodontic dentistry.

Intraseptal Injection

A sharp fine needle is inserted in between teeth into the septal bone. Once the needle is within the bone the anesthetic solution is injected slowly. The solution diffuses through the cancellous bone to anesthetize the nerve at the periapical region. The advantage of this method is that, the anesthesia of the tooth is achieved without anesthetizing the surrounding tissues. As the injection causes certain amount of pain and as there are chances of needle breakage, this method is not in practice.

Intraligamental Injection

In this technique, the solution is deposited directly into the periodontal membrane. A fine gauge needle is inserted between the bone and the tooth (Fig. 5-7). The solution then should be deposited very slowly. The solution infiltrates through the periodontal tissues and anesthetizes the nerve at the periapical region of the tooth. Profound anesthesia of the tooth may be achieved

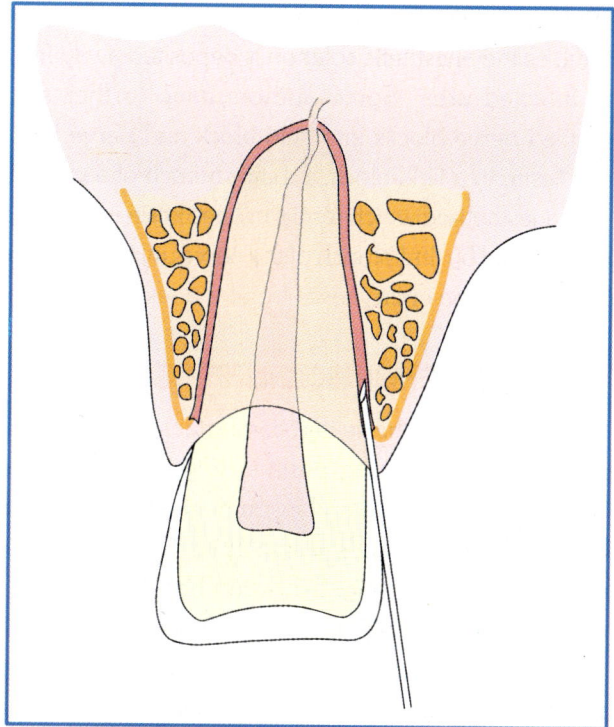

Fig. 5-7: Diagrammatic representation of intraligamentary injection

without anesthesia of surrounding tissues. The disadvantage in this case is that the forcible injection which may cause pain and sometimes, the tooth may extrude slightly from the socket. As the injection is made through the gingival crevice, it may facilitate the infection to spread into the periodontal membrane. Hence prior to the injection, the sulcus of the tooth should be cleansed thoroughly with an antiseptic solution.

Nerve Block Anesthesia

Anesthesia can be achieved in the entire region supplied by the nerve when anesthetic solution is deposited close to the major nerve trunk. In nerve block anesthesia, the needle is inserted further into the tissues to reach the area of the main nerve trunk. In the process of inserting the needle deeper into the tissues, there is every chance of a blood vessel being pierced or a nerve being injured. Such complications can be minimized if a proper technique is followed and certain precautions taken during injection. In case of infection in relation to periapical region of a tooth, block anesthesia would be useful, as the anesthetic solution is deposited away from the infected area. Some authors have further sub-classified nerve blocks into field block and nerve block anesthesia. In a field block, a major branch of a nerve is being anesthetized which results in anesthesia in a limited field supplied by that branch of the nerve unlike the nerve block, where the entire nerve trunk is anesthetized.

PRECAUTIONS BEFORE LOCAL ANESTHESIA

The patient should be seated comfortably in the dental chair in a semi-reclining position (Fig. 5-8). It is also necessary that injection and instruments should be kept away from the patient's vision (Figs 5-9 and 5-10). Loading the syringe (Fig. 5-11) and handling of dental instruments (Fig. 5-12) in front of the patient should be avoided. The dental surgeon should also learn to carryout all dental procedures in a sitting position. The area of needle insertion in the oral cavity should be coated with an antiseptic solution. Excess of antiseptic solution should be wiped from the area. Application of surface anesthetic at the point of needle insertion is important to prevent pain during insertion of the needle. After the injection the patient should be under constant observation. A casual conversation with the patient

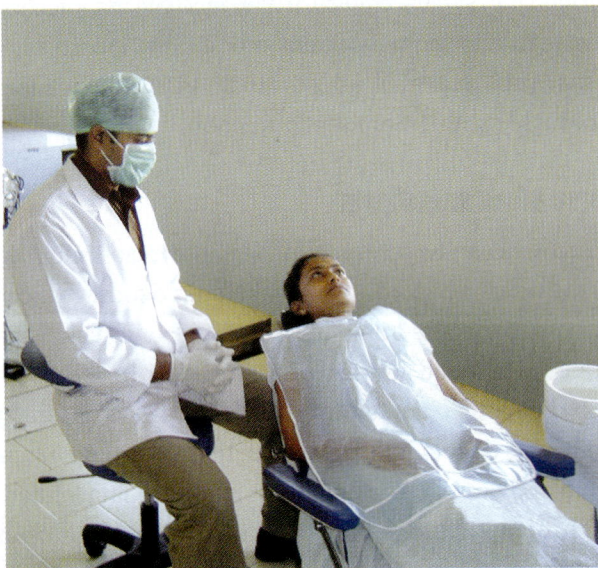
Fig. 5-9: Syringe being loaded behind the patient or away from the patient's vision

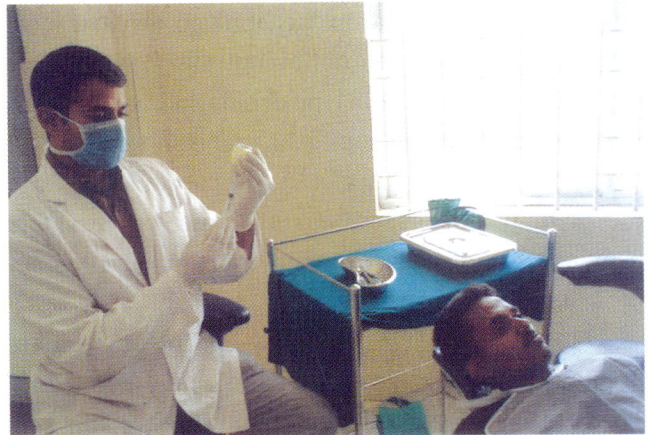
Fig. 5-10: Instruments being handled from the back of the patient, away from patient's vision which is ideal

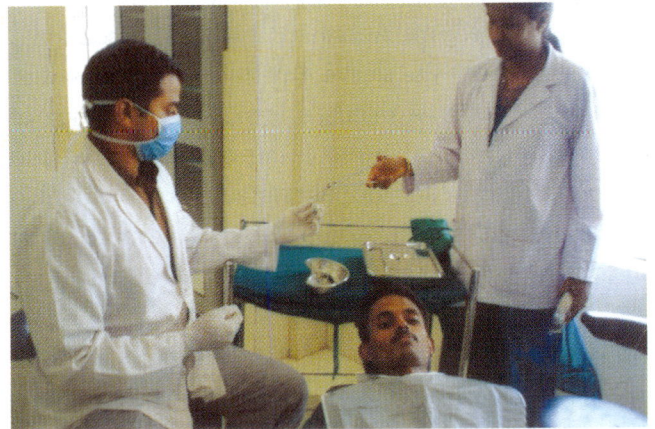
Fig. 5-8: Comfortable position of the patient in the dental chair and the ideal sitting position of the operator

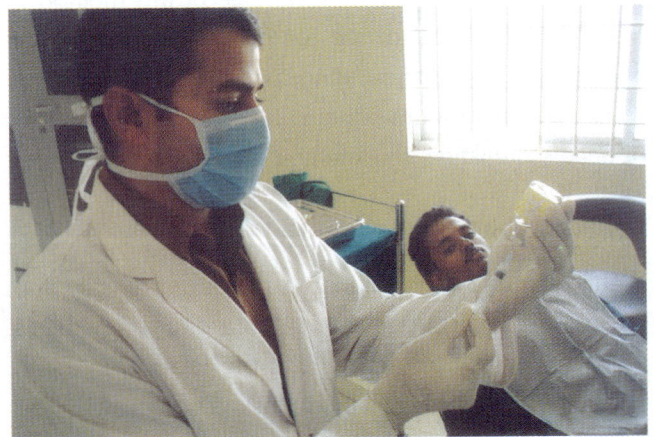
Fig. 5-11: Syringe being loaded in front of patient's vision. This should not be done as it will cause psychological fear in the mind of the patient

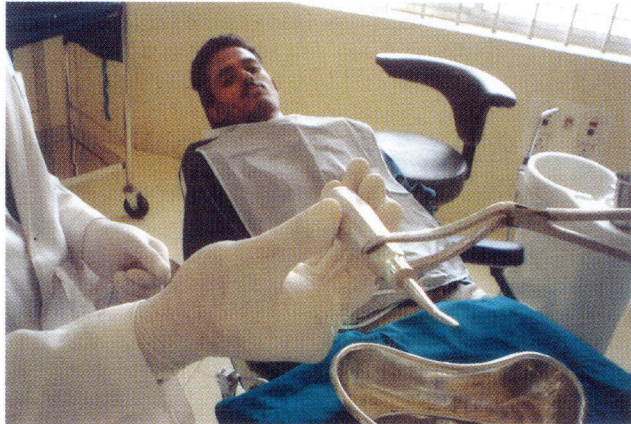

Fig. 5-12: Instruments being handled in front of the patient's vision results in anxiety and fear. This should not be practiced

especially if the patient is a child will ally fear and anxiety of patients. After a waiting period of 5 minutes the anesthetic action should be tested by questioning the patient about effect of anesthesia. Patient may express that there is numbness, swelling in the area or no pain in that particular tooth. Apart from this clinically absence of pain can be elicited with a sharp probe on the mucous membrane in the anesthetized area.

6 | Armamentarium

To administer local anesthesia, essential requirements are a syringe, a needle and the anesthetic agent.

SYRINGES

Charles Gabriel Pravaz in 1853 designed an all-metal hypodermic syringe to administer certain drugs. At about the same time Alexander Wood designed a glass and metal syringe to administer drugs subcutaneously. Later in 1912 Dr. Thew designed a high-pressure syringe. It was only in 1917, due to the efforts of Harvey S Cook the cartridge system of loading syringes was adopted. Prior to manufacture of anesthetic cartridges the anesthetic solution used to be drawn into the metal or glass syringes. With the availability of anesthetic cartridges many types of cartridge syringes were designed and considerable improvement occurred over the years.

Different Cartridge Syringes Available

1. Reusable metal syringe—top loading—non-aspirating type (Fig. 6-1).

   The main disadvantage in this type of syringe is the aspiration cannot be done and the operator would not know whether an intravascular deposition of anesthetic solution has been made during routine administration of local anesthesia.

2. Reusable metal syringe—top loading—aspirating type (Figs 6-2A to F).

   Aspirating syringes are popular since one can easily make out in case the needle has entered a

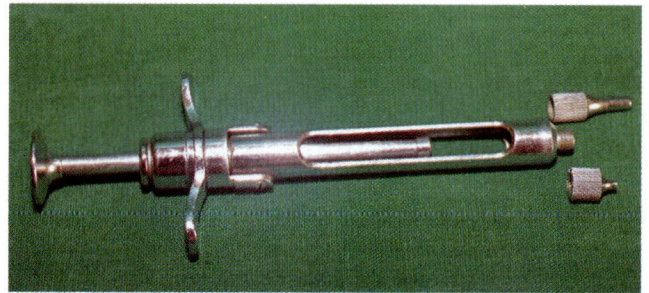

Fig. 6-1: A non-aspirating type of metal cartridge syringe with two types of hubs. Short hub is for shorter needle and the longer one for the longer needle. The non-aspirating type of syringe is at present not in use

blood vessel. During aspiration if no blood is drawn into a syringe the anesthetic solution can be safely deposited into the tissues.

3. Reusable metal syringes – breach loading – aspirating type.

   Here the cartridges are loaded from one side of the syringe.

4. Reusable metal syringes – breach loading – self-aspirating type.

   Aspiration of a syringe is desirable before depositing anesthetic solution if one wants to avoid accidental intravascular injections. In the above type of syringe the plunger is pressed on the rubber bung before depositing the solution. The elasticity of the bung creates a positive pressure within the cartridge. Once the pressure on the plunger is released there is negative pressure within the cartridge which results in automatic aspiration.

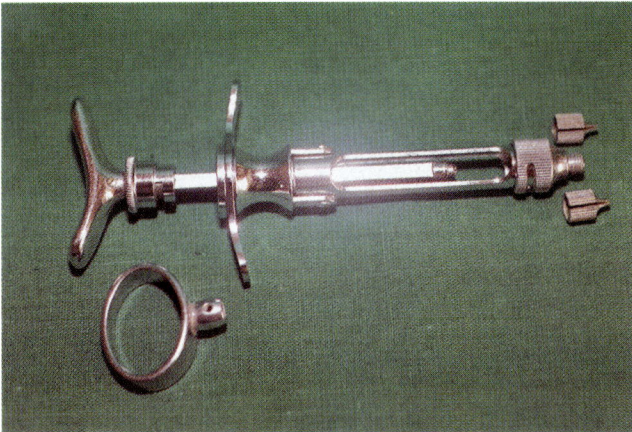

Fig. 6-2A: An aspirating type of metal cartridge syringe along with separate thumb holder and modified hubs

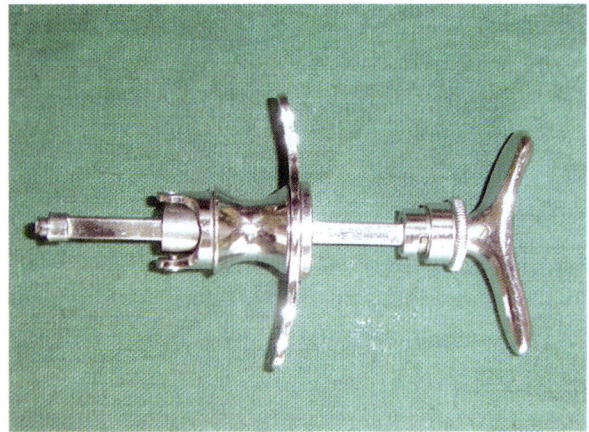

Fig. 6-2B: Plunger part of the cartridge syringe. Note at the tip of the plunger barbs which engage the rubber bung in a open position. This can be closed or opened by turning the knob at the handle region. Engaging the rubber bung in cartridge helps in aspiration

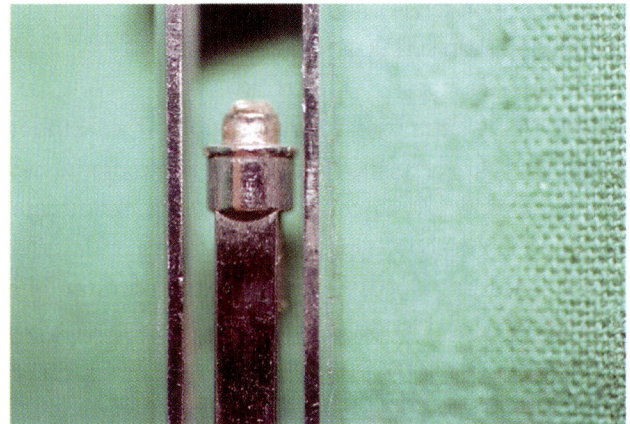

Fig. 6-2C: End of the plunger—enlarged view showing the barbs in open position

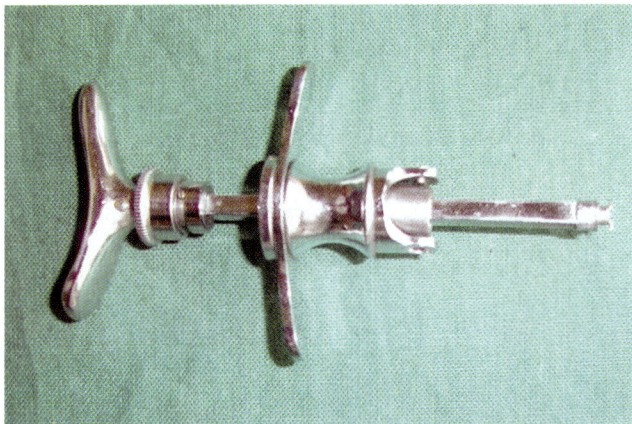

Fig. 6-2D: Plunger part of the cartridge syringe. Note at the tip of the plunger the barbs are in closed position

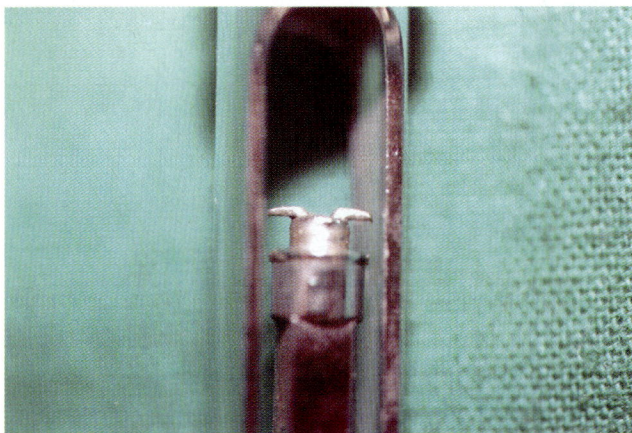

Fig. 6-2E: End of the plunger—enlarged view showing the barbs in closed position

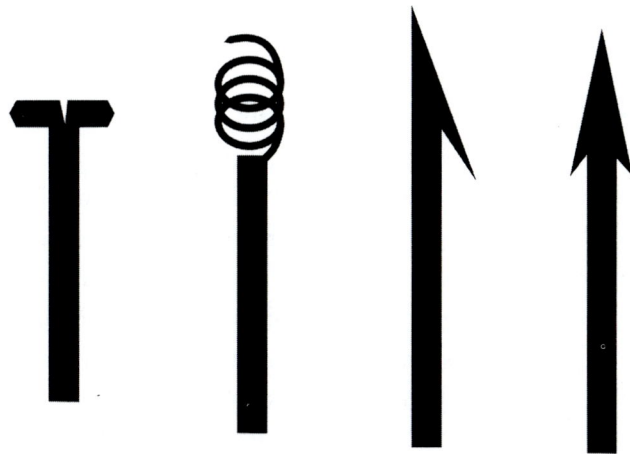

Fig. 6-2F: Different types of plunger tips for engaging the rubber bung in the anesthetic cartridge

5. Reusable plastic syringe – breach loading - aspirating type – for cartridges.

   This syringe is similar to the metal type except that it is less expensive and lightweight.

6. Disposable plastic syringes for cartridges – aspirating type.

   Any armamentarium used in medical or dental field, if it is disposable, the patients in general, accept it without any doubts. The disadvantage is the cost involved.

Apart from the regular cartridge syringes some more types of syringes have been designed to make the deposition of anesthetic solution much easier.

1. Power operated syringes
2. Spring driven syringes
3. Pressure syringes

In certain situations for deposition of anesthetic solution the plunger of the syringe need to be compressed with force especially in case of palatal and periodontal injections. In the above types of syringes the manual force is not required. The Wilcox–Jeroett obtunder, the pressure injector was developed in 1905 specifically for periodontal injections. From then many more syringes for intraligamentary injection was designed and modified for easy handling of the syringes. Eitrajet, Ligmaject and Peripress are some of the later improved versions of syringes for intraligamentary injections. Due to high cost of these syringes, these are not routinely used in this country.

Development of Syringes in India

In India glass syringes with metal pistons and later, all glass syringes in Luer Mount and Luer-Lok types (Fig. 6-3A and B) were used in both medical and dental field. Stainless steel needles were used along with these syringes. Both syringe and needle were repeatedly used after sterilization. The anesthetic solution was drawn from multidose vials. This frequent use of same syringes and needles lead to post-injection infection in many cases.

Use of cartridge syringes for anesthetic cartridges were introduced during 70's. Though it became popular for a

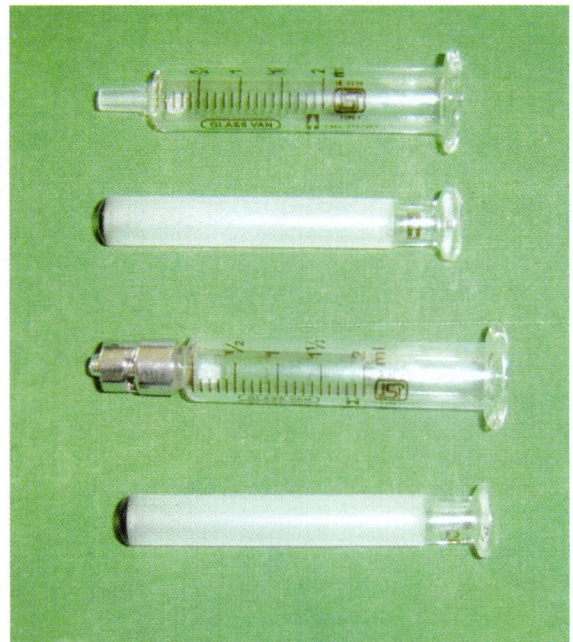

Fig. 6-3A: Glass syringe (2 ml)-Luer Mount and Luer-Lok types

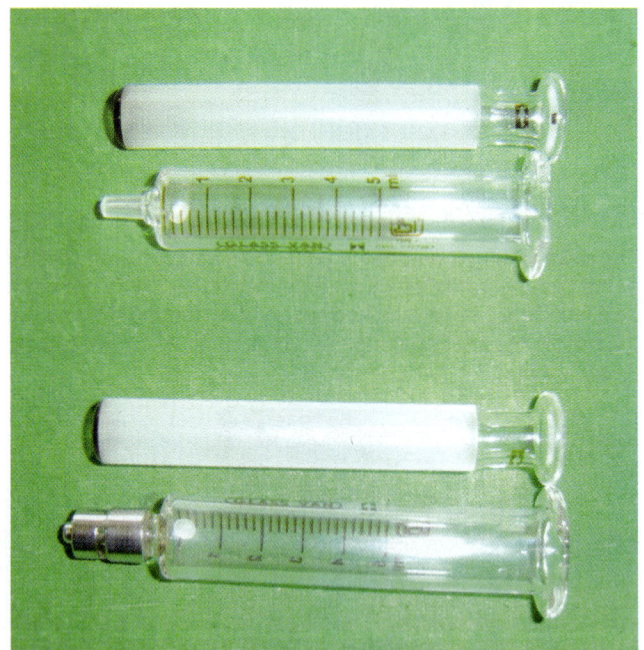

Fig. 6-3B: Glass syringe (5 ml)-Luer Mount and Luer-Lok types

brief period of time it was given up because of the cost factor. At the same time disposable plastic syringes came into usage and gained popularity (Figs 6-4A and B). The disposable plastic syringes are being extensively used

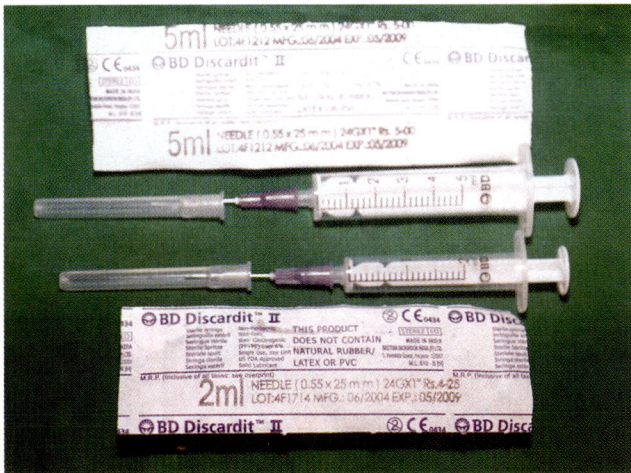

Fig. 6-4A: Disposable (2 ml and 5 ml) plastic syringes with their sterile packing—Luer Mount type

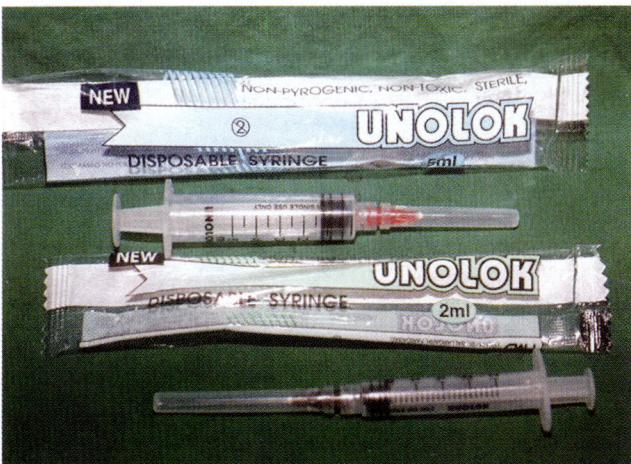

Fig. 6-4B: Disposable (2 ml and 5 ml) plastic syringes with their sterile packing—Luer-Lok type

by the medical and dental professionals. The popularity of its use is due to the fact that it is one time use and cost effective. People could afford it. More importantly patients in general accepted it as a safe method. Due to increase in awareness of HIV and AIDS infection people started demanding use of disposable syringes and needles. Some patients doubting the use of disposables started bringing the syringes along with them. Many a time doctors and dental surgeons had to open the sealed packing of syringes in front of the patient. The increase use of disposable syringes triggered more manufacturers

to come into the field. This reduced the cost of syringes further. Today more than 98% of doctors and dental surgeons use disposable plastic syringes in their practice.

Jet Injectors

The first jet injector in dentistry was used in 1958 by Margetis and associates. Syrijet mark II and Panjet injectors have been used in western countries. These injectors do not contain any needle and the anesthetic agent is delivered in spray form under pressure. This results in instant penetration of the anesthetic solution through the skin or the mucous membrane. The spray has to be directed perpendicular to the surface. Improper handling of the equipment will result in injury to the mucous membrane. Although Mada-jet a jet injector is being marketed in India, due to high cost it is not in routine use.

Computer Aided Delivery System

The first computer controlled local anesthetic delivery system (CCLAD) was introduced into dentistry in 1997. This system consists of a lightweight handpiece mounted with a fine needle connected to the cartridge by a fine flexible cannula. The cartridge is mounted on the system. The insertion of the needle, the force of the injection and the amount of solution delivered is completely controlled by computer operation. This results in minimum discomfort to the patient and reduces the pain to a great extent compared to manually operated cartridge syringes. Several brands of CCLAD such as Wand/Compudent, Quick sleeper and Anaeject are available in USA, Europe and Japan. The only disadvantage probably is the cost factor.

NEEDLES

Needles are required to administer anesthetic solution from a syringe. With the development of different types of syringes, needles have also undergone many improvements.

Different Types of Needles

Reusable Steel Needles for Cartridge Syringes (Figs 6-5A and B)

These needles are mounted on the cartridge syringe and fixed in place by the use of a hub. Different hubs are available for different applications.

The shorter end of the needle is for piercing the diaphragm of the anesthetic cartridge when it is loaded into the syringe. Reusable needles were used several times, each time after sterilization. The disadvantage was that the needles used to get damaged at their tips during mounting and fixing. Small modification of the hub was made to avoid placing the hub from the top (Figs 6-5C and D). The other disadvantages were difficulty in

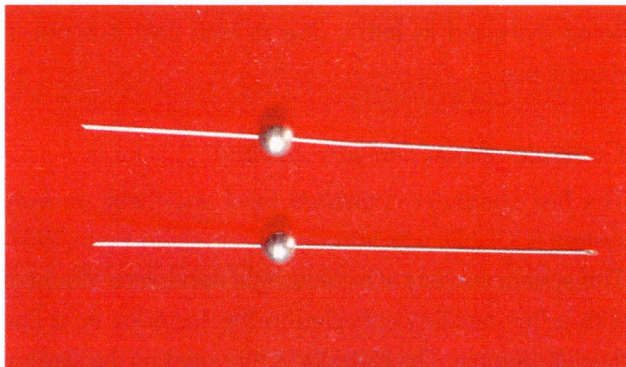

Fig. 6-5C: Hub being introduced from the top to fix the needle in position

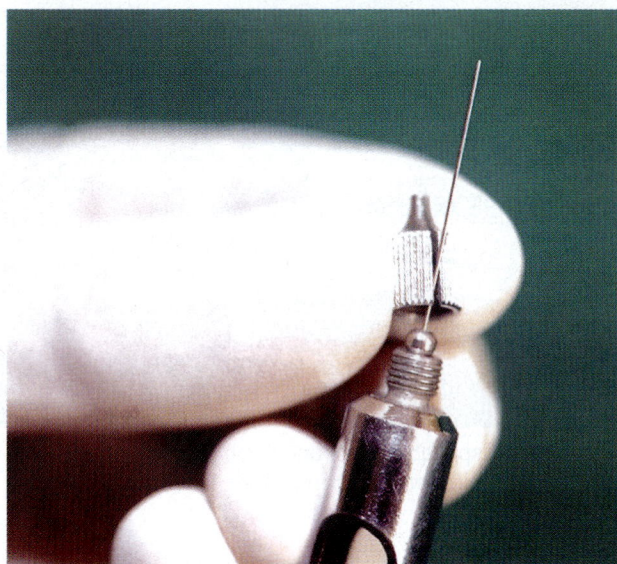

Fig. 6-5A: Reusable needles for cartridge syringe. They were repeatedly used after sterilization. They are no longer in use

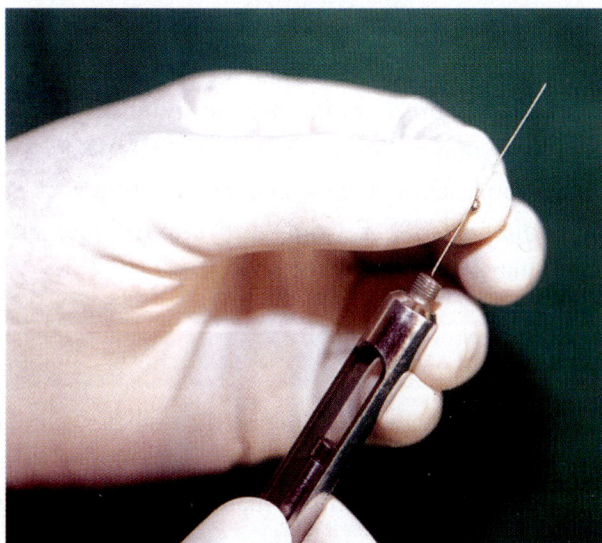

Fig. 6-5D: Modified hub being introduced from the side

sterilization and blunting of needles. Moreover repeated use of same needle was not accepted. These needles are no longer in use.

Disposable Stainless Steel Needles with Attached Plastic Hub (Figs 6-6A and B)

This was a great improvement over the reusable needles. These needles are available in individual pre-sterilized packing and are meant for single use. This is now being routinely used by the majority of dental surgeons.

Fig. 6-5B: Reusable needle being introduced into the cartridge syringe

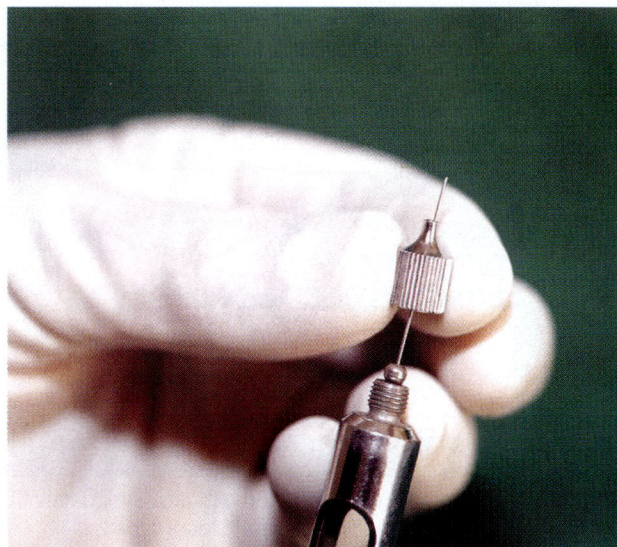

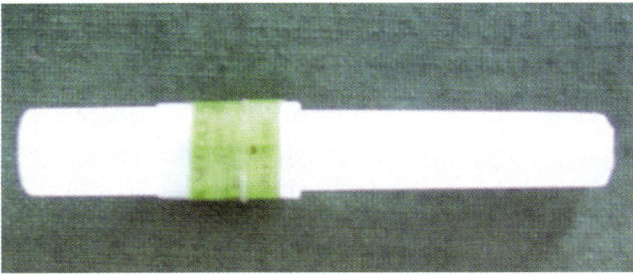

Fig. 6-6A: Disposable needle for cartridge syringe in its sterile packing

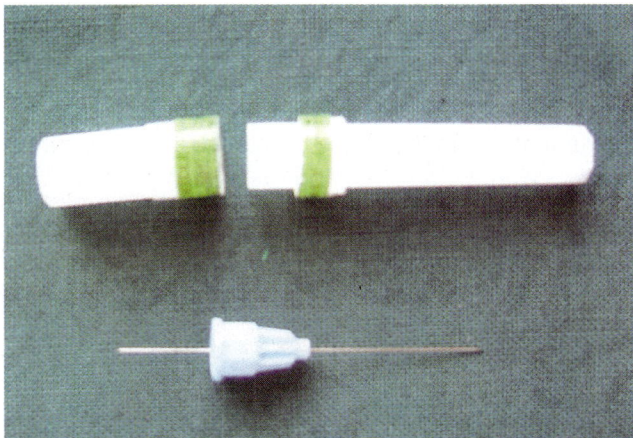

Fig. 6-6B: Disposable needle with a fixed plastic hub removed from the sterile packing

Disposable Cartridge Mounted Needle

Here handling of the needle was minimal. The cartridge and the needle were available in presterilized packing. This only required a special type of syringe.

Disposable Syringe with Mounted Needle with Safety Covering (Fig. 6-7A)

Safety plus is a sterile, disposable, reloadable auto-aspirating integrated injection system a product from Septodont company (Fig. 6-7B). Here the syringe and the mounted needle is readily available in a sterile form. The cartridge is loaded into the syringe and the plunger is attached to the cartridge. The needle cap is removed just before injection. Once the solution is deposited the safety covering automatically slides over the needle thus protecting the doctor or the assistant from needle injuries during handling.

Septodont have also introduced safety plus with metal handle accessory and also a handle for

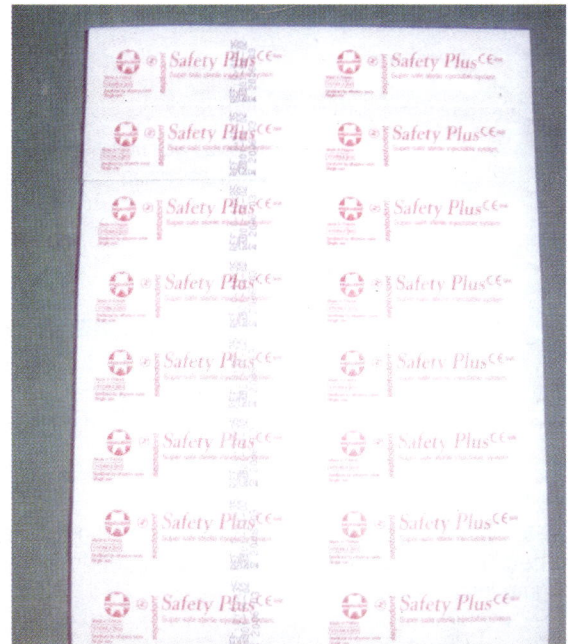

Fig. 6-7A: Safety syringe with needle in its sterile packing

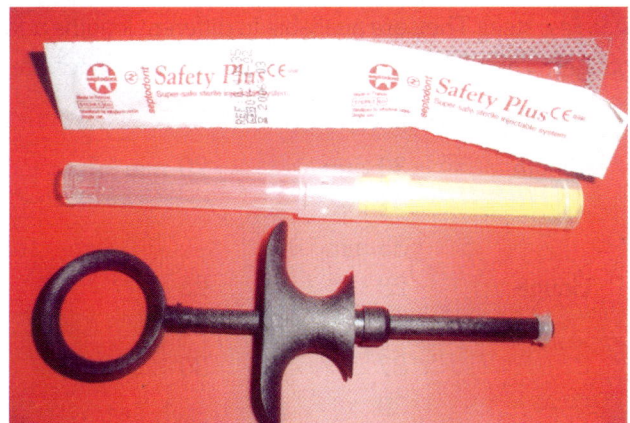

Fig. 6-7B: Safety syringe with mounted needle with needle covering and plunger which is to be attached to the cartridge is also seen

intraligamentary injections (Fig. 6-8). These syringes have not been introduced in Indian market because of the cost factor.

Disposable Loaded Syringe with Mounted Needle and the Syringe Preloaded with the Anesthetic Agent

This would be ideal for a dental surgeon as there is no handling of needle or cartridge, a totally ready to use armamentarium for local anesthesia in dentistry.

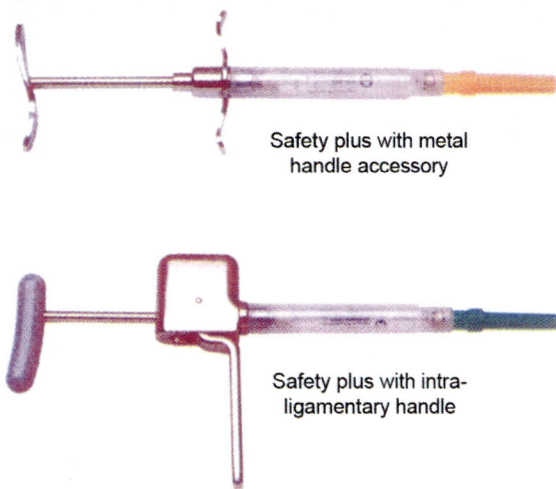

Safety plus with metal handle accessory

Safety plus with intra-ligamentary handle

Fig. 6-8: Shows safety plus syringe with mounted needle and attached metal handle and the other syringe with intraligamentary handle

All the needles used in dentistry are made from stainless steel. They are available in different lengths and gauges. The commonly used needles for cartridges are:

Needles	Long	Short
Length	30 mm	20 mm
	32 mm	
	35 mm	
Gauge	23	25
	25	27
	27	30
	30	

The long needles are used for block anesthesia and shorter needles for infiltration anesthesia. The most common gauge of needle in practice in western countries is 25. The above needles are available in presterilized ready to use packings.

In India during 50's and 60's reusable stainless steel needles (Fig. 6-9) were used along with reusable glass syringes. In 70's disposable syringe and needles gained popularity and is being used routinely. The needles are made of stainless steel and the mounted hub is made of plastic.

Different length and gauges of the needles are available. The packing and the hub of the needle is color

coded (Figs 6-10A and B). The commonly used needles in dentistry in this country are:

Needles	Long	Short	Short
Length	38 mm	25 mm	12 mm
	(1½ inches)	(1 inch)	(½ inch)
Gauge	26	22	26
		23	
		24	

The needle and syringes after its use have to be properly disposed of to avoid misuse and reuse. The needles can be disposed of in special containers for sharp instruments. In India needle burners and syringe cutters

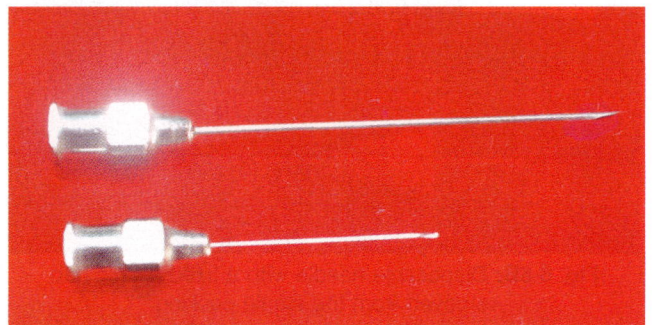

Fig. 6-9: Reusable steel needles. These were being used along with reusable glass syringes after repeated sterilization. These are no more in use

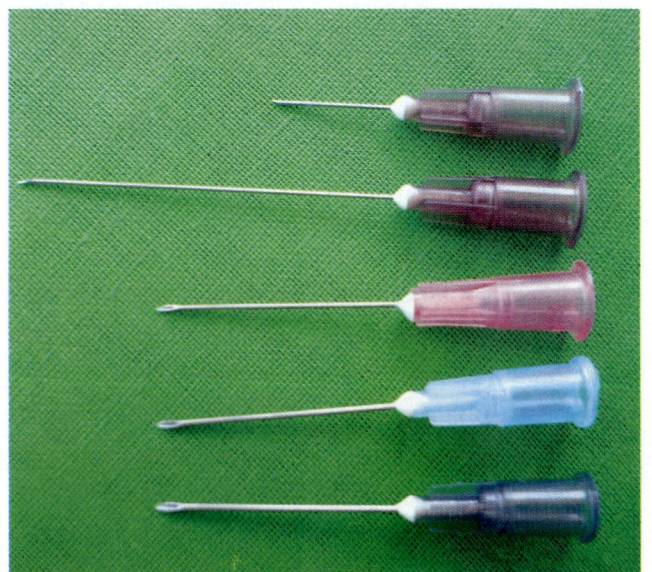

Fig. 6-10A: Disposable needles with plastic hub-from top-1' x 22, 1' x 23, 1' x 24, 1 ½ ' x 26 and ½' x 26. These are colour' coded

Fig. 6-10B: Same disposable needles in their sterile packing

Fig. 6-10D: Tip of the needle viewed from front—Note the bevel of the needle tip

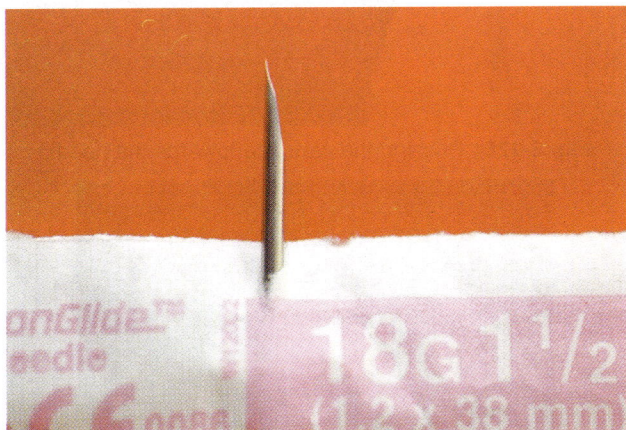

Fig. 6-10C: Tip of a needle viewed from side

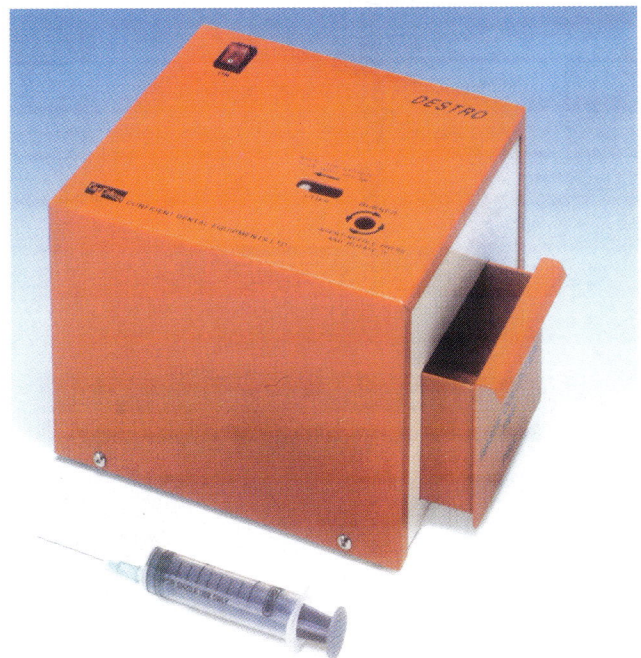

Fig. 6-11A: Needle burner cum syringe cutter

are available for use in clinics and hospitals (Figs 6-11A and B).

These are not expensive and dental surgeons should start using them in their clinics.

ANESTHETIC SOLUTION

Anesthetic solution in cartridges for use along with cartridge syringes are available in 1.8 ml, 2.0 ml and 2.2 ml. In India 2.0 ml cartridges of lignocaine are available. The cartridges are glass tubes sealed at one

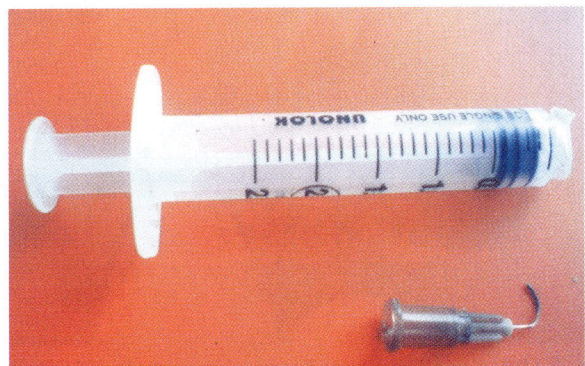

Fig. 6-11B: Burnt needle and the cut hub of syringe

end by a diaphragm partially covered by alluminium cap. The opposite end of the cartridge is sealed with a rubber bung which can be moved down the cartridge with a cartridge syringe plunger (Fig. 6-12A). Before loading the cartridge in the syringe the surface of the diaphragm needs to be wiped with 70% ethyl alcohol to disinfect the surface diaphragm (Fig. 6-12B). The cartridge when loaded into the syringe, is slightly and

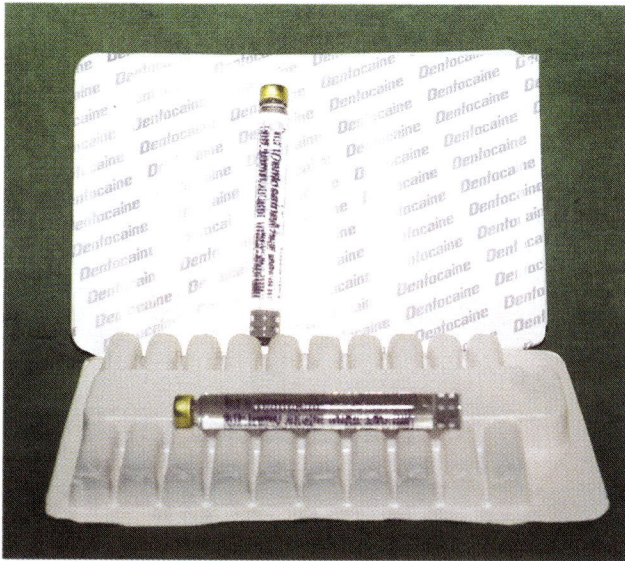

Fig. 6-12C: Loading the syringe with the anesthetic cartridge

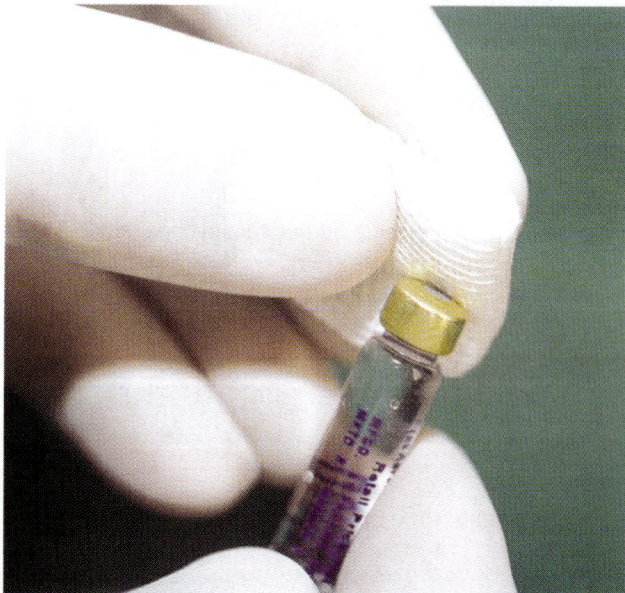

Fig. 6-12A: Anesthetic cartridge with sterile packing

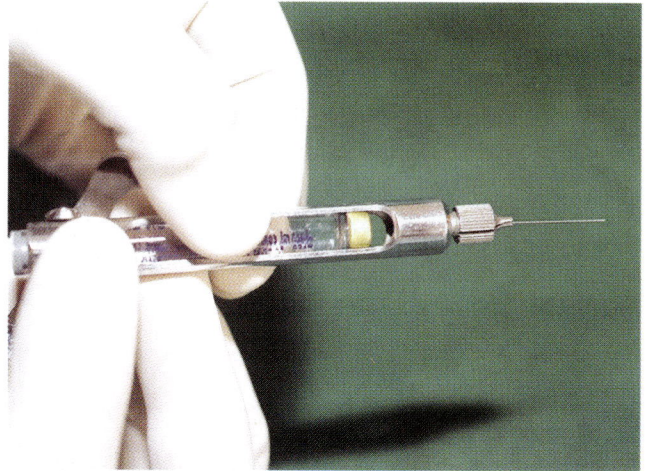

Fig. 6-12D: Pushing the cartridge towards the needle

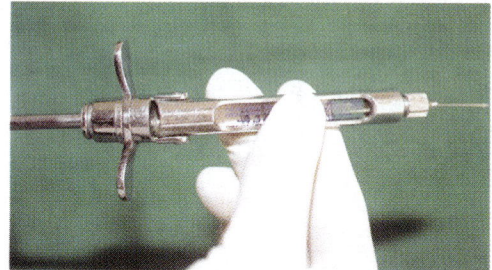

Fig. 6-12E: Closing the plunger into place

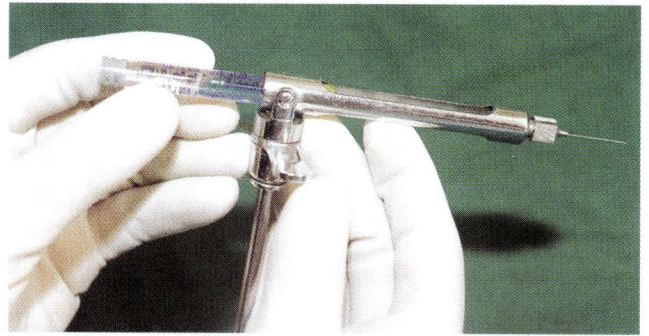

Fig. 6-12B: Anesthetic cartridge-diaphragm being disinfected by wiping the surface with 70% ethyl alcohol

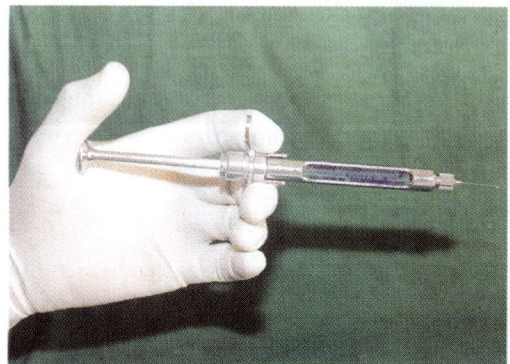

Fig. 6-12F: Syringe ready for injection

firmly pushed down with finger so that the shorter end of the needle pierces the cartridge through the diaphragm (Figs 6-12C and D). Now position the plunger and a gentle push is made on the rubber bung to remove the air from the needle (Figs 6.12E and F) and to confirm that the needle is not blocked. The syringe is now ready to be used for intraoral injection.

The anesthetic cartridges available in USA mostly contain 1.8 ml of anesthetic drug. The different types of anesthetics used in USA are:

Lidocaine, Xylocaine, Octocaine, Alphacaine — Lidocaine 2% with epinephrine { 1: 50,000 / 1: 100,000 } — Lidocaine 2% without epinephrine

Polocaine, Carbocaine, Scandnest — Mepivacaine 3% without vasoconstrictor / Mepivacaine 3% with levonordefrin 1: 20,000

Citanest — Prilocaine 4% plain / Prilocaine 4% with epinephrine 1:200,000

Septocaine — Articaine 4% with epinephrine 1:100,000 / Articaine 4% with epinephrine 1:200,000

Mascaine — Bupivacaine 0.5% with epinephrine 1:200,000.

Anesthetic Drugs Available in India

There are very few pharmaceutical companies manufacturing local anesthetic products for dental anesthesia. Lignocaine is the most popular anesthetic agent used in both dental and medical practice. Apart from this Bupivacaine is more popularly used in medical practice. The use of bupivacaine a long acting anesthetic in Dental practice is very minimal. These anesthetic drugs are available in multidose vials. Each vial consists of 30 ml except sensarcaine vials which contains 20 ml of solution The manufacturers recommend maximum of 10 withdrawals since frequent piercing of the rubber diaphragm may contaminate the solution.

1. *Xylocaine 2% with adrenaline 1:200,000 (Fig. 6-13)*

Each ml contains:

Lignocaine hydrochloride IP	21.3 mg
Adrenaline	0.005 mg
(as Adrenaline bitartrate) IP	
Sodium chloride	6.0 mg
Sodium metabisulphite	0.5 mg
Methylparaben	1.0 mg

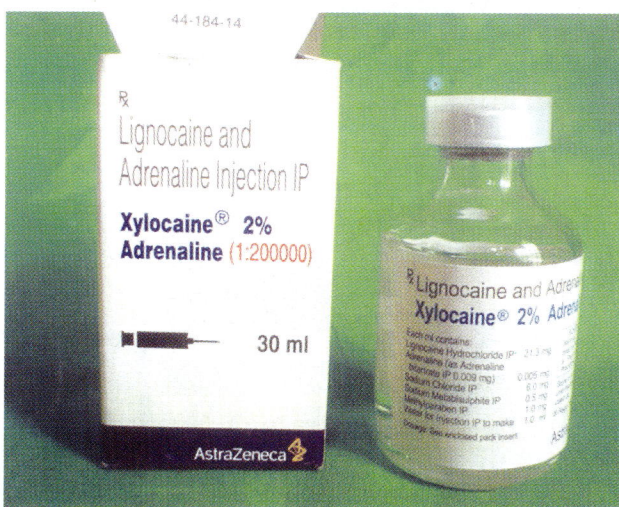

Fig. 6-13: Xylocaine 2% solution with adrenaline 30 ml multidose vial

Table 6.1: Multidose vials of anesthetic solution			
Product name	Generic name	Vasoconstrictor	Manufacturer
Xylocaine 2% with adrenaline	Lignocaine Hydrochloride	Adrenaline 1: 200,000	Astra Zeneca
Xylocaine 2%	Lignocaine Hydrochloride	—	Astra Zeneca
Lignox 2% A	Lignocaine Hydrochloride	Adrenaline 1:80,000	Waren Pharmaceuticals
Lignox 2%	Lignocaine Hydrochloride	—	Waren Pharmaceuticals
L-caine 2%	Lignocaine Hydrochloride	Adrenaline 1: 80,000	Group Pharmaceuticals
Sensarcaine 0.5%	Bupivacaine	—	Astra Zeneca

Water for injection IP to make   1.0 ml

Maximum individual dose – not to exceed 4.5 mg / kg body weight.

Total maximum dosage – not to exceed 200 mg (in an adult of 70 kg)

2. *Xylocaine 2% (Fig. 6-14)*

Each ml contains :

Lignocaine hydrochloride IP		21.3 mg
Sodium chloride	IP	6.0 mg
Methylparaben	IP	1.0 mg

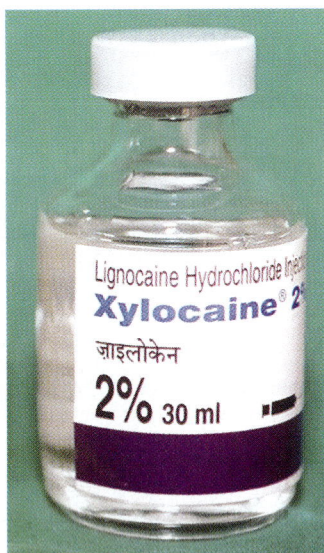

Fig. 6-14: Xylocaine 2% solution (plain) 30 ml multidose vial

Water for injection IP to make   1.0 ml

3. *Lignox 2% A with adrenaline 1:80,000 (Fig. 6-15)*

Each ml contains :

Lignocaine hydrochloride IP		24.64 mg
Adrenaline	IP	0.0125 mg
Methylparaben	IP	1.0 mg
Propylparaben	IP	0.5 mg
Water for injection	IP	QS

4. *Lignox 2% (Fig. 6-16)*

Each ml contains :

Lignocaine hydrochloride IP		20.0 mg
Methylparaben	IP	1.0 mg
Propylparaben	IP	0.5 mg
Water for injection	IP	QS

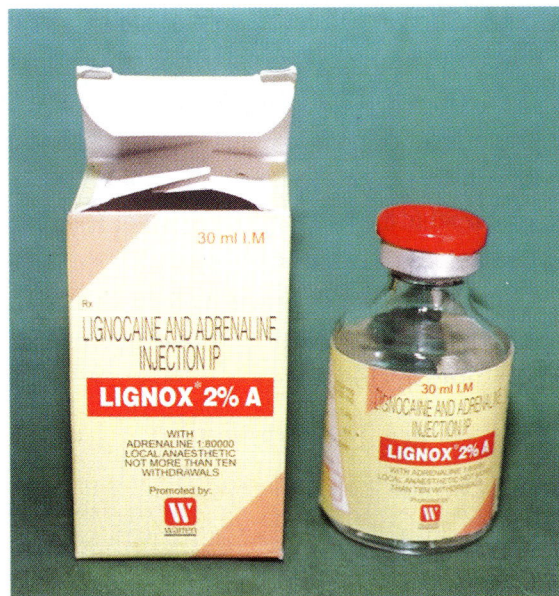

Fig. 6-15: Lignox 2% with adrenaline—30 ml multidose vial

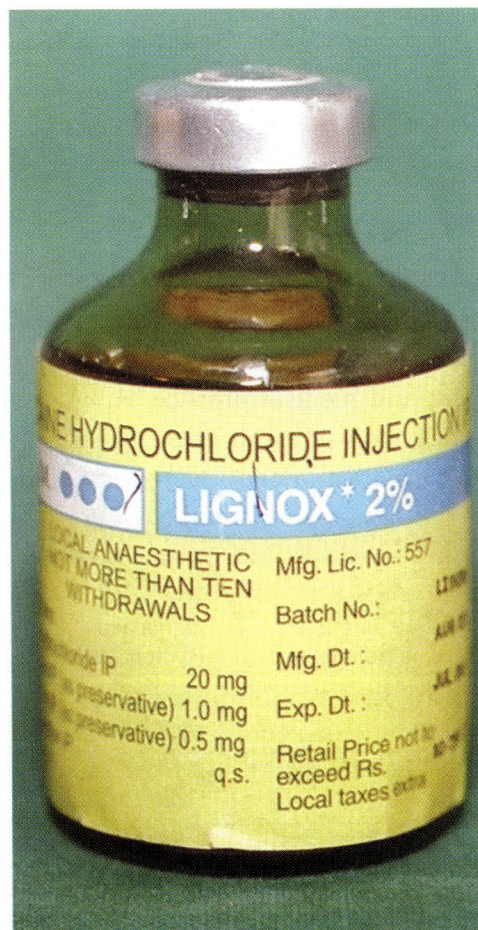

Fig. 6-16: Lignox 2% (plain)—30 ml multidose vial

5. *L-Caine 2% A with adrenaline 1:80,000 (Fig. 6-17)*
   Each ml contains :

Lignocaine hydrochloride	IP	24.64 mg
Adrenaline	IP	0.0125 mg
(as Adrenaline bitartrate)	IP	
Sodium metabisulphite	IP	1.0 mg
Propylparaben	IP	0.5 mg
Water for injection		QS

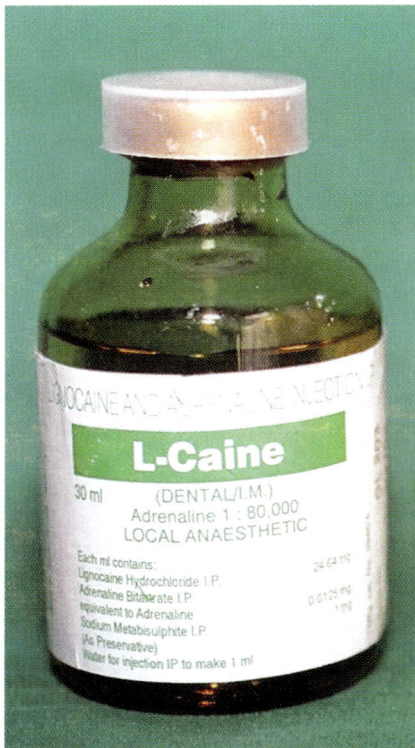

Fig. 6-17: L-Caine 2% with adrenaline—30 ml multidose vial

6. *Sensorcaine 0.5 % (Fig. 6-18)*
   Each ml contains :

Bupivacaine HCL (anhydrous)	USP	5.0 mg
Sodium chloride	IP	8.0 mg
Methylparaben	IP	1.0 mg
Water for injection	IP to make	1.0 ml.

Sensorcaine injections are available 0.25% and 0.5% strengths. Sensorcaine 0.25% is recommended for lengthy oral surgical procedures. Sensorcaine 0.5% injections can be used for spinal anesthesia in surgeries

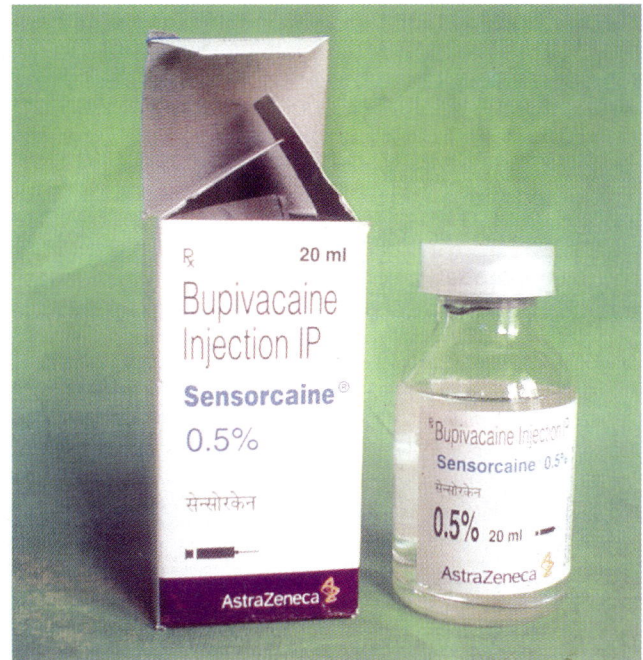

Fig. 6-18: Sensorcaine 0.5%

lasting 2 to 2.5 hours. Bupivacaine cartridges manufactured in the name of marcaine contains 0.5% with 1:200,000 epinephrine. This has been recommended in lengthy oral surgical procedures. Sensorcaine available in India does not contain any vasoconstrictors. Excessive plasma levels might reach with higher dosage.

Ointments, Jelly and Viscous

1. *Xylocaine 5% - ointment (Astra Zeneca) (Fig. 6-19)*
   Contents:

Lidocaine	USP	5% w/w
Propelene glycol	IP	25% w/w
Ointment base	QS	

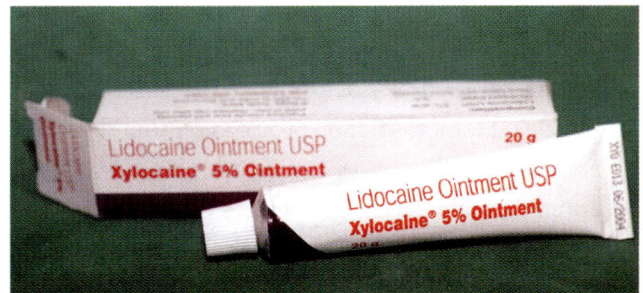

Fig. 6-19: Xylocaine 5% ointment

Xylocaine ointment contains 5% lignocaine base in a vehicle consisting of carbowaxes and propylene glycol available in 10 gm and 20 gm packings.

2. *Xylocaine 2% gelly (Astra Zeneca) (Fig. 6-20)*
   Composition:

Lignocaine hydrochloride	IP	2.0% w/v
Methylparaben	IP	0.061% w/v
Propylparaben	IP	0.027% w/v
Water soluble gel base in purified water		QS

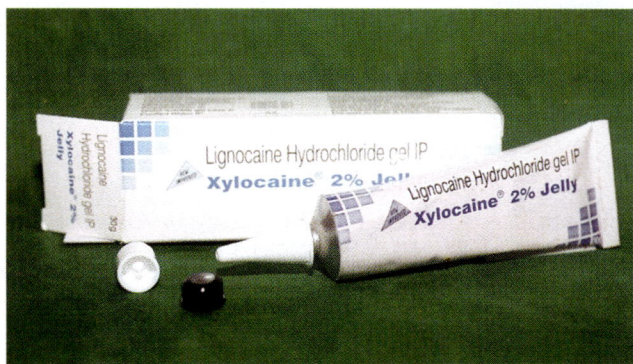

Fig. 6-20: Xylocaine 2% gelly

The xylocaine gelly is a water miscible base, characterized by high viscosity and low surface tension, brings the anesthetic into intimate contact with tissues. Anesthesia usually occurs rapidly within 5 minutes and gives effective anesthesia for nearly 20-30 minutes. Available in 30 gm tubes. It is frequently used during nasoendotracheal introduction, catheterization, gastroscopy, and bronchoscopy.

3. *Xylocaine – Topical solution 4% (Astra Zeneca)*
   Each ml contains – Lignocaine hydrochloride 42.7 mg.
   Methyl parahydroxy benzoate – as preservative.
   Xylocaine topical solution provides profound surface anesthesia within 1 to 5 minutes and persists for approximately 15 to 30 minutes. Absorption from wound surfaces and mucous membrane is relatively high. Flow of solution in the oropharyngeal region may interfere in swallowing.

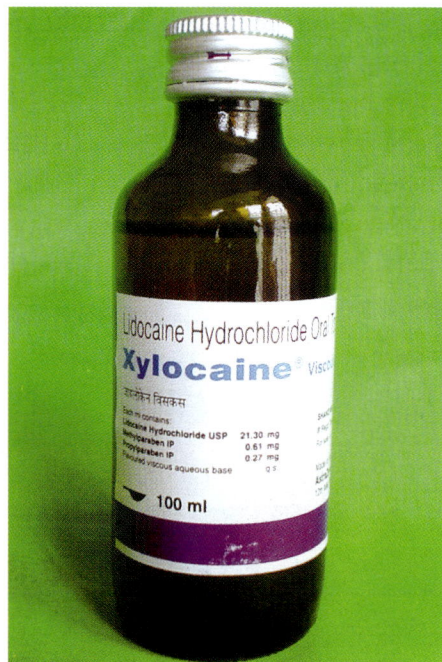

Fig. 6-21: Xylocaine 5% viscous

4. *Xylocaine Viscous 2% (Astra Zeneca) (Fig. 6-21)*
   Each ml contains :

Lignocaine hydrochloride	IP	21.3 mg
Methylparaben	IP	0.61 mg
Propylparaben	IP	0.27 mg
Flavored viscous aqueous base		QS

   Because of low surface tension the xylocaine viscous comes into intimate contact with the surface of the mucous membrane and the viscosity ensures prolonged contact with the surface prolonging the action.

Aerosal Sprays

1. *Xylocaine 10% spray – Lidocaine topical aerosol (Astra Zeneca) (Fig. 6-22)*
   Each ml contains:

Lidocaine	USP -	100 mg
Ethanol	IP	28.29% v/v.

   The anesthesia usually occurs within 1 to 5 minutes and persists for 10 to 15 minutes. Each activation of the metered dose delivers 10 mg of lignocaine base.

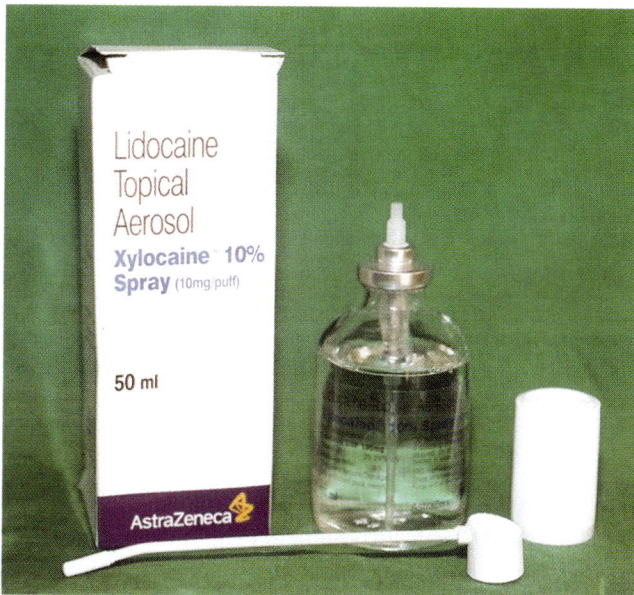

Fig. 6-22: Xylocaine 10% aerosol spray

According to the manufacturer it is unnecessary to dry the site prior to application. It is available in 50 ml packing.

2. *Lignox 10% spray – Lidocaine topical aerosol (Waren) (Fig. 6-23)*

Each ml contains:

Lidocaine USP 15% w/w

Flavored vehicle and propellant QS to 100% w/w

Each metered dose delivers – Lidocaine USP 7.5 mg

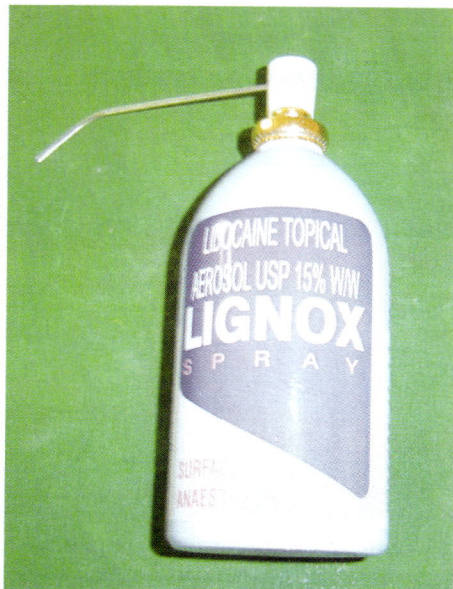

Fig. 6-23: Lignox 10% aerosol spray

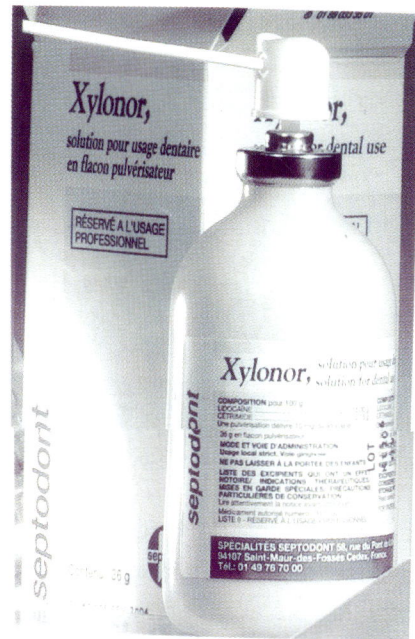

Fig. 6-24: Xylonor spray a surface anesthetic

3. *Xylonor spray—topical aerosol (Septodont) (Fig. 6-24)*

Composition—per metered dose

Lidocaine base	10.00 mg
Centrimide	0.10 mg
(as a disinfectant)	
Excipients	Saccharin, natural mint flavor,
	Dipropylene glycol,
	ethylic alcohol at 95% (v/v)

Few other aerosol local anesthetic sprays available are Nummit and Orikains.

Anesthetic Cartridges

1. Dentocaine – 2 ml cartridges – 2% E.80 (Muller and Phipps (India) with adrenaline 1 : 80,000 (6-25).

   Each ml contains:

Lignocaine hydrochloride		24.64 mg
Adrenaline	IP	0.0125 mg
Thymol	IP	0.40 mg
Chlorobutol (as preservative)		5.00 mg
Ringer's solution	USP	0.29 ml
Water for inj.	IP	to make 1.00 ml

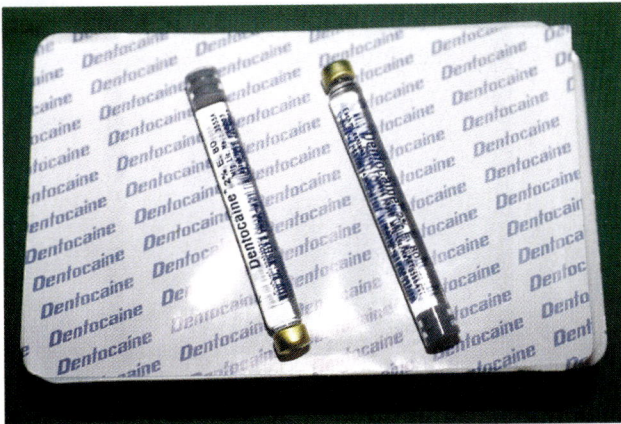

Fig. 6-25: Anesthetic cartridge 2 % Dentocaine

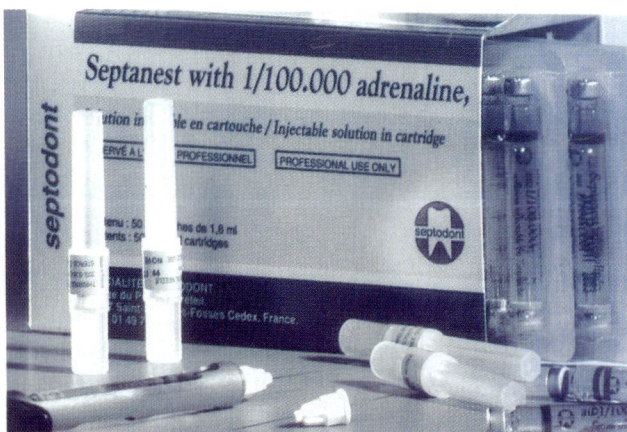

Fig. 6-27: Cartridge packing of spetanest with adrenaline 1:200,000 in its sterile packing

2. Septodont company have recently introduced in Indian market many of their anesthetic products. All these products are available in cartridge form.

   a. *Septanest – 4% Articaine HCl in 1.7 ml cartridges with adrenaline – 1: 100,000 (Fig. 6-26)*

   Contents – (per cartridge)

Articaine hydrochloride (INN)	68.000 mg
Epinephrine bitartrate (INN)	30.94 micrograms
Adrenaline tartrate	17.00 micrograms
(expressed in base)	(1: 100,000)

   Excipients—Sodium chloride, Sodium metabisulphite, Sodium hydroxide solution, water for Injection.

   Anesthesia by infiltration and block anesthesia is achieved in 2 to 5 minutes.

Septanest 4% is also made available with adrenaline in 1: 200,000 concentration (Fig. 6-27)

Contents – (per cartridge)

Articaine hydrochloride (INN)	68.000 mg
Epinephrine bitartrate (INN)	15.47 micrograms
Adrenaline tartrate	8.50 micrograms
(expressed in base)	(1: 200000)

   Excipients—Sodium chloride, Sodium metabisulphite, Sodium hydroxide solution, water for Injection.

   b. *Lignospan 2% special – 2% Lidocaine with adrenaline (Fig. 6-28)*

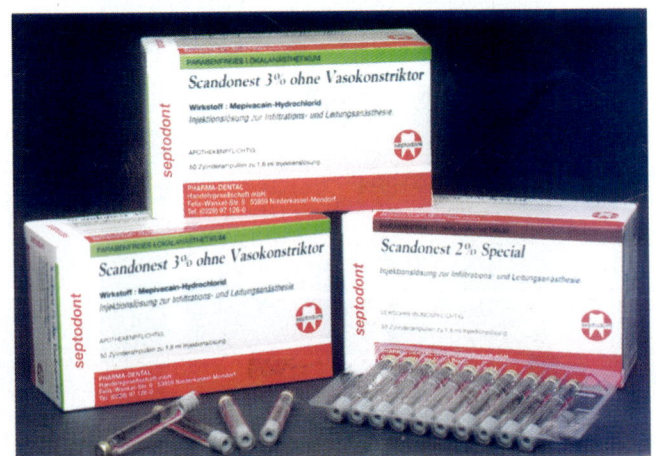

Fig. 6-26: Cartridge packing of septanest with adrenaline 1:100,000 cartridges in its sterile packing

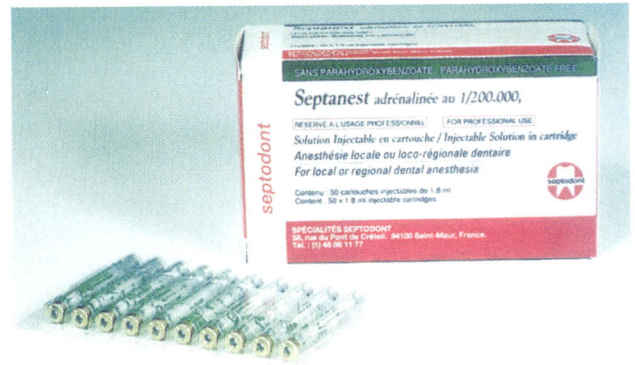

Fig. 6-28: Cartridge packing of scandonest 3% without adrenaline and scandonest 2% special in their sterile packings. Notice the depression in the rubber bung for attachment of the plunger

Contents –

Lignospan (INN) hydrochloride	- 36 mg
Adrenaline tartrate	- 22.5 mg
Isotonic solution ad	- 1.8 ml

c. *Scandones 3% plain – 3% Mepivacaine hydrochloride (Fig. 6-29)*

Contents:

Mepivacaine Hydrochloride	- 66 mg
Water for injection ad	- 2.2 ml

This has a rapid onset of anesthesia and acts for a short duration 20 to 30 minutes. Available in 2.2 ml autoinjectable cartridges.

d. *Scandonest 2% special – 2% Mepivacaine hydrochloride with adrenaline in 1:100,000.*

Contents :

Mepivacaine hydrochloride	- 66 mg
Adrenaline (INN) base	- 1:100 000
Water for injection ad	- 2.2 ml

It has rapid onset of action but prolonged action.

Available in 2.2 ml autoinjectable cartridges.

Apart from these there are no other known manufacturers of cartridges in India. There may be few other firms and the products have not been listed in medical formulation publications.

The multidose vials are supplied in sealed packings. The seal should be broken (Fig. 6-29) and the rubber cap should be disinfected by wiping with a gauze piece soaked in 70% ethyl alcohol (Fig. 6-30). Anesthetic solution from the multidose vials are withdrawn into a syringe whenever it is required. To avoid frequent piercing of the rubber cap a 22 gauge 1-inch needle can be pierced into the rubber cap (Figs 6-31 and 6-32). Whenever anesthetic solution is required the syringe can be attached to the needle in the vial and required amount of solution withdrawn (Figs 6-33 to 6-35). The syringe is detached and the needle is left behind in the vial. For injections a separate needle (1 inch 24 gauge or 1½ inch 26 gauge) is attached to the

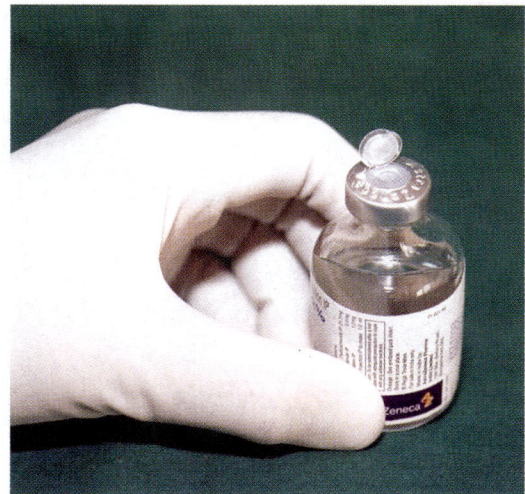

Fig. 6-29: An anesthetic vial being kept ready for withdrawing the solution. Note the circle on the rubber stopper where the needle insertion is made

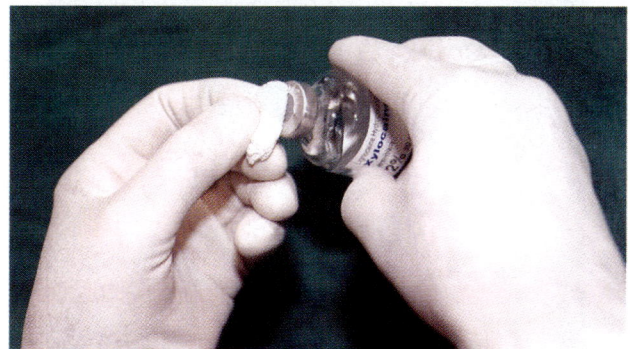

Fig. 6-30: Rubber cap of the anesthetic vial being wiped with a sterile gauze soaked in 70% ethyl alcohol. This is to disinfect the area of needle insertion

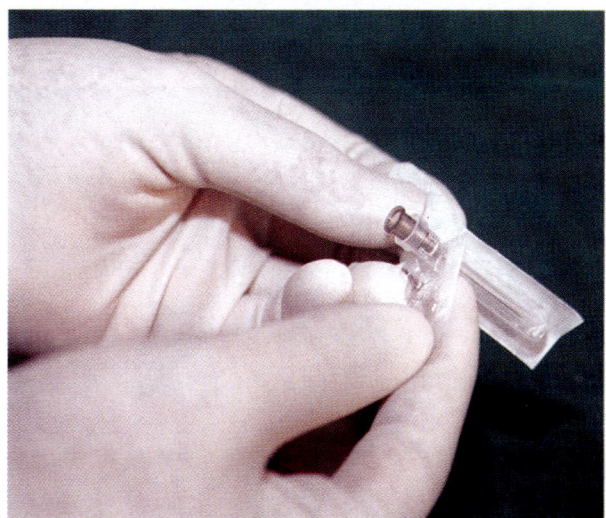

Fig. 6-31: A sterile packing being opened to pick up the needle with needle cover

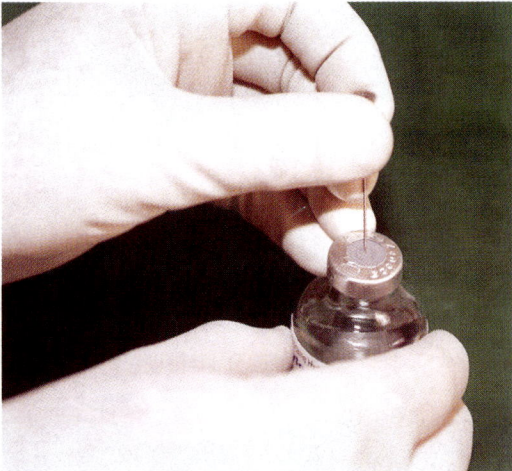

Fig. 6-32: A one inch 22 gauge needle being inserted into the multidose vial

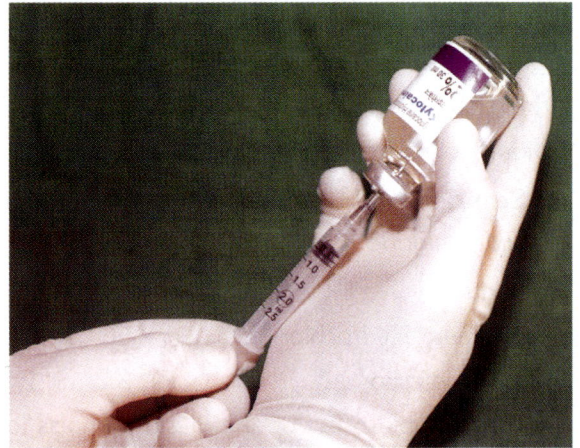

Fig. 6-33: A disposable syringe being taken out of a sterile packing

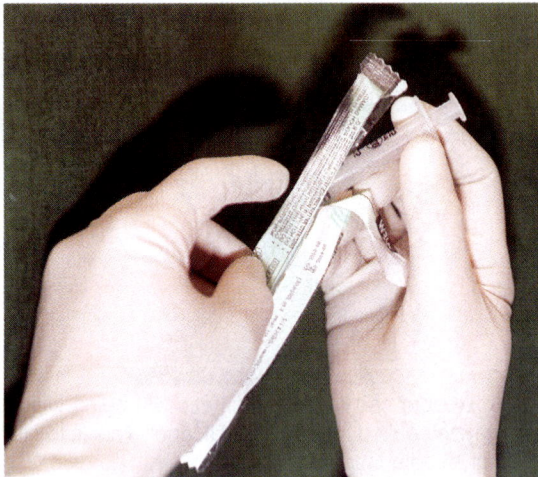

Fig. 6-34: The 2 ml syringe being attached to the needle which is a luer loc attachment

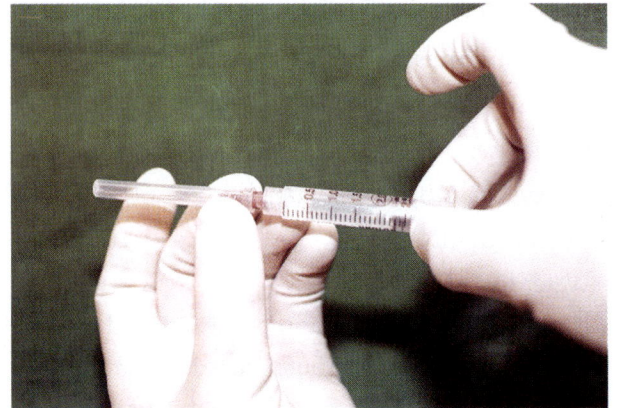

Fig. 6-35: Anesthetic solution being withdrawn from a vial

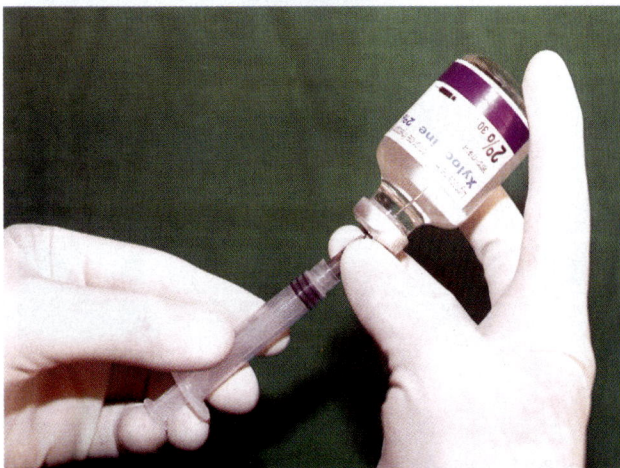

Fig. 6-36: A separate sterile 1 ½ inch 26 gauge needle being attached to the loaded syringe

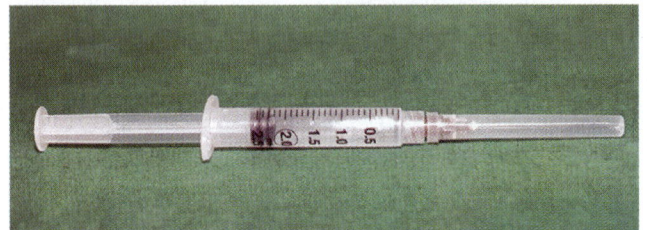

Fig. 6-37: The loaded syringe kept ready for injection

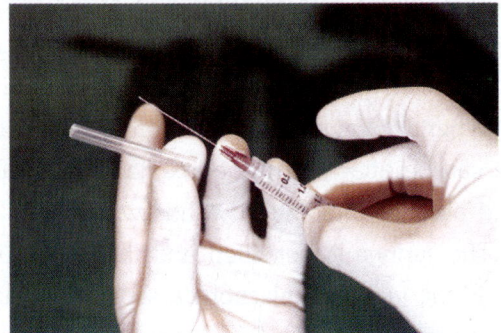

Fig. 6-38: The needle cover being removed just before injection

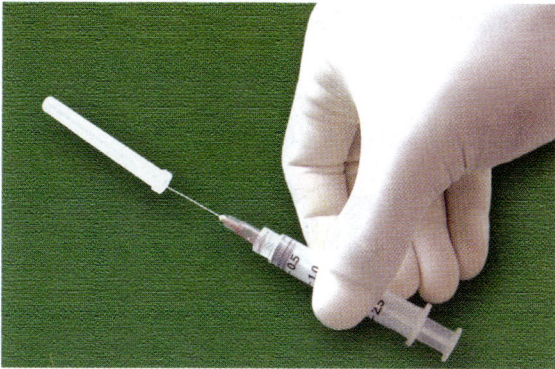

Fig. 6-39: Needle is being caped after the injection

syringe (Figs 6.36 and 6.37). Immediately after the use the needle should be caped to avoid any needle injury (Figs 6.38 and 6.39).

This procedure can be followed in a hospital or a dental clinic, where there is frequent usage of anesthetic injections. In case the anesthetic solution is not frequently used it is better to use a fresh needle to withdraw the solution each time it is required. The needle and syringe after use should be destroyed properly.

7 Local Anesthesia in Maxillary Region

The maxillary alveolar bone covering the roots of the teeth is porous and the cortical plate is very thin. The roots of the teeth are close to the surface of the bone. It is only in the region of the root of zygoma that the cortical bone is thick and non-porous (Fig. 7-1). The porous nature of the maxillary bone is favourable for anesthetic solution to diffuse through the bone into the periapical region of teeth. For extractions of maxillary teeth except 1st molar, infiltration anesthesia can be satisfactorily employed.

METHOD OF INFILTRATION ANESTHESIA

When the patient comfortably seated, the cheek is retracted with a mouth mirror or fingers to give a clear view of the mucobuccal fold. The area of needle

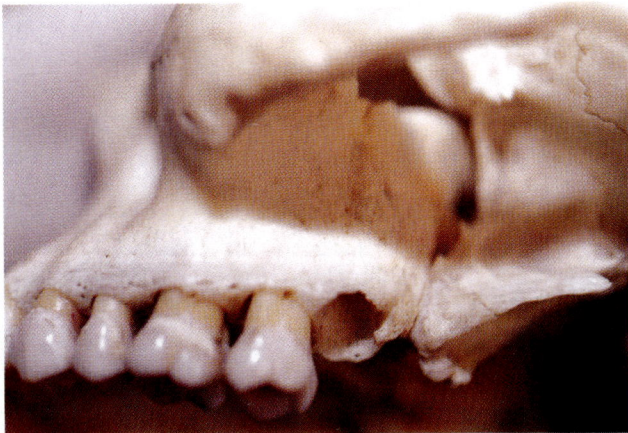

Fig. 7-1: Shows maxillary alveolar bone being porous. Note the thick alveolar bone at the periapical region of the 1st molar. Here the bone is not porous

insertion is dried with a sterile swab (Fig. 7-2A) and a suitable antiseptic solution is applied over the region (Fig. 7-2B). Excess of antiseptic solution should be taken out with a sterile swab (Fig. 7-2C). Now a surface anesthetic is applied with a cotton bud (Fig. 7-2D) to minimize the pain during needle insertion.

The syringe loaded with the anesthetic solution is held in pen grasp. The syringe and the needle should be placed at 20° angulations to the buccal bone (Fig. 7-3A). The needle is then inserted into the mucous membrane, approximately at the periapical region of the tooth (Fig. 7-3B) to be anesthetized. The needle is inserted upto 2 to 3 mm deep, upto the periosteum. The syringe should be aspirated before depositing the solution. For infiltration anesthesia of a single tooth, about one ml of the solution is deposited slowly. Fast deposition of the solution results in pain and should be avoided. In cases where two or three teeth are to be anesthetized, the syringe is slightly withdrawn and is inserted towards the periapical region of the next tooth. Aspiration should again be done before deposition of the solution. The process can be repeated to the neighboring tooth on the opposite side. In this way anesthesia of 2 or 3 teeth can be accomplished from a single point of needle insertion. For anesthetizing the upper central incisor, after depositing the required amount of solution at the periapical region of the particular incisor tooth, the needle is slightly withdrawn and directed towards the neighboring central incisor

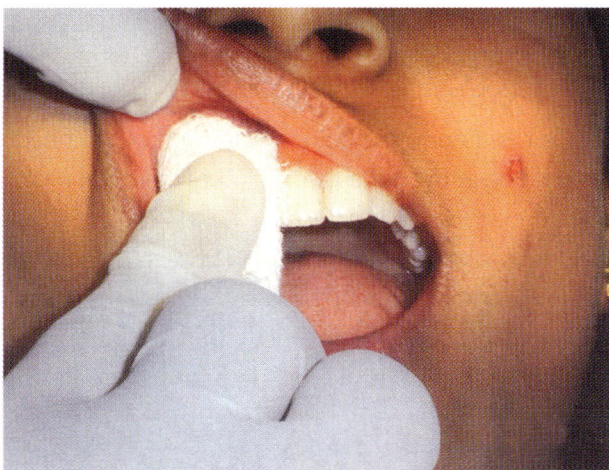

Fig. 7-2A: Wiping the surface of mucous membrane at the site of needle insertion with a sterile swab

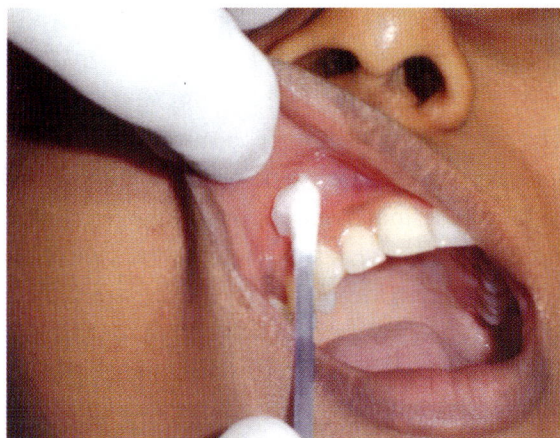

Fig. 7-2B: Applying antiseptic solution at the place of needle insertion

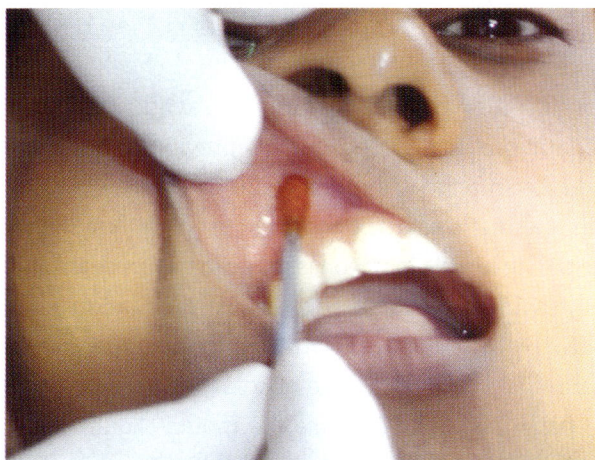

Fig. 7-2C: Removing the excess of antiseptic liquid with sterile swab

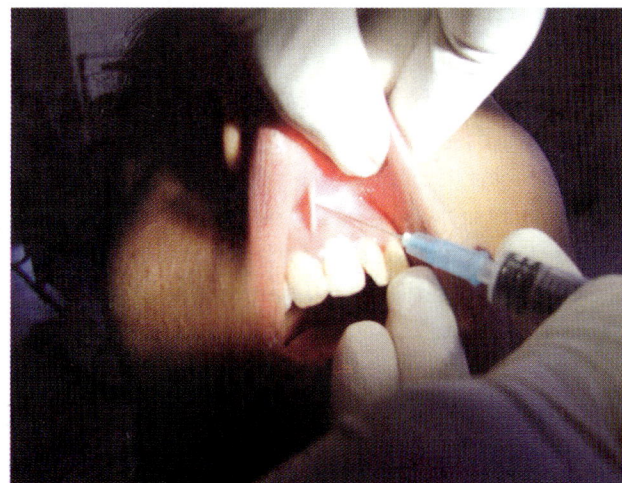

Fig. 7-2D: Applying surface anesthetic (ointment) at the point of needle insertion.

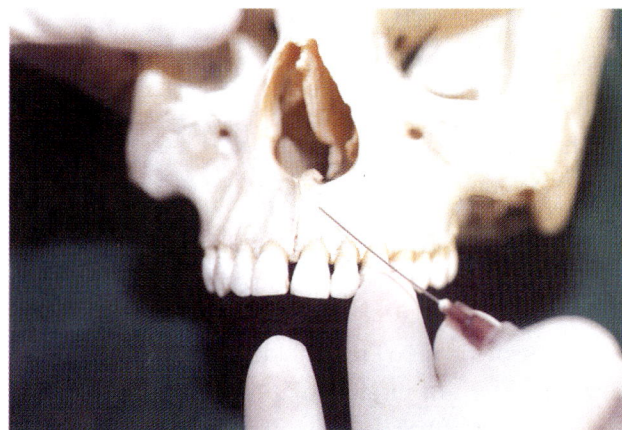

Fig. 7-3A: Position of the needle for infiltration anesthesia in the periapical region on the labial region of the left upper central incisor. Note the porosity of bone in this region

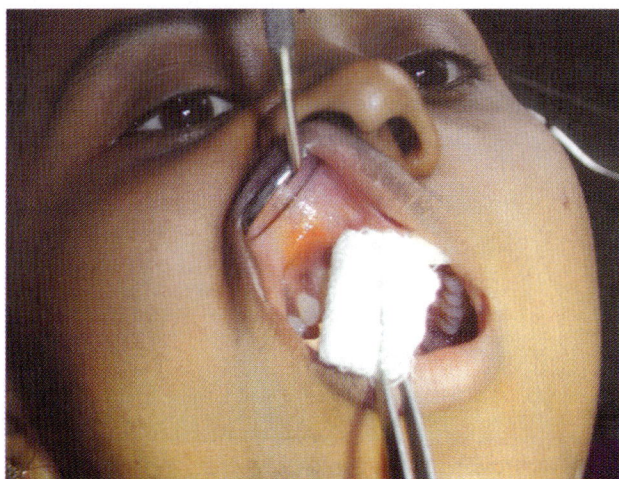

Fig. 7-3B: Position of the needle for infiltration anesthesia of the left central incisor being demonstrated in a patient

crossing the midline. Half cc of solution should be deposited in this position to anesthetize nerve fibers crisscrossing the midline.

The three molar teeth in the maxilla can be conveniently anesthetized by a posterior superior alveolar nerve block anesthesia, except the mesiobuccal root of the 1st molar tooth. For anesthetizing the mesiobuccal root of 1st molar, a few drops of the solution are deposited in the periapical region of that root. The 2nd and 3rd molar teeth can also be effectively anesthetized by infiltration anesthesia, as the tuberosity of the maxilla is quite porous in nature.

By injecting anesthetic solution supraperiosteally on the labial or buccal aspect, in addition to the tooth, the alveolar bone, periosteum and the mucous membrane in that region can be anesthetized. For the removal of teeth the palatal mucous membrane has to be anesthetized by a separate injection as it is supplied by greater palatine and nasopalatine nerves (see palatal injection).

POSTERIOR SUPERIOR ALVEOLAR NERVE BLOCK

This is one of the many nerve blocks, frequently used in dentistry. The anesthetic solution in this method is deposited behind the tuberosity, near the posterior superior alveolar nerve before it enters the maxillary sinus. This is also termed as tuberosity block. To effectively anesthetize the posterior superior alveolar nerve, the following landmarks should be carefully assessed.

1. The position of the tuberosity of maxilla should be palpated by the index finger. Sometimes when the third molar has not erupted or has been removed, the tuberosity will be placed much further backwards than the distal surface of the 2nd molar. In cases where the third molar is absent, the tuberosity position will be distal to the 2nd molar tooth. As the needle has to be inserted along the surface of tuberosity, it is important to visualize and palpate the position of tuberosity.

2. The point of insertion of the needle for administring this nerve block is approximately the periapical region

of the distal root of 2nd molar (Fig. 7-4A). This point is considered when the third molar is erupted, embedded or has been removed. In case the third molar is absent, the point of insertion of the needle would be at the periapical region of the distal root of 1st molar tooth.

3. Root of zygoma is the junction between maxilla and the zygomatic bone. The alveolar bone is slightly thicker and curves outwardly in this region.

The region should be palpated to assess its position.

Technique of Injection

The patient should be comfortably seated in a semi-reclining position. The operator sits in the right front position. The cheek is retracted with a cheek retractor, mouth mirror or finger of the left hand. Preliminary preparations are carried out (as previously explained) and a 2cc syringe with 1½ inch 26 gauge needle loaded with anesthetic solution is held in the right hand in pen grasp. The needle insertion is made at the predetermined point with the syringe kept at 30° angulation to the buccal plate and at 45° angulation to the upper occlusal plane (Fig. 7.4B). Once the needle is close to the bone, the patient is asked to close the mouth slightly. As the needle is inserted further into the tissue, close to the bone, the syringe is swung on to the lateral aspect, to

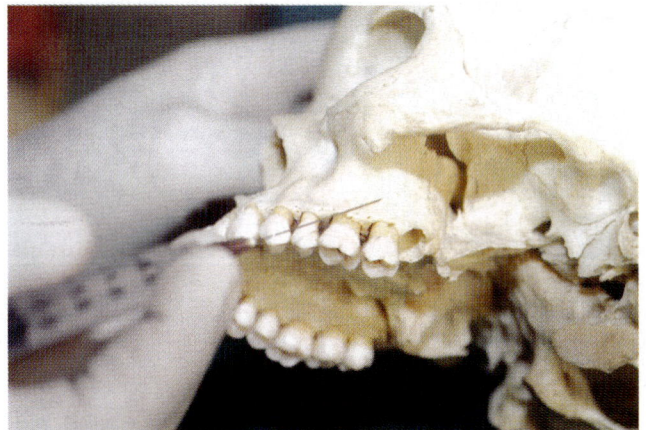

Fig. 7-4A: Position of the needle while inserting the needle for a posterior superior alveolar nerve block anesthesia demonstrated on the maxilla

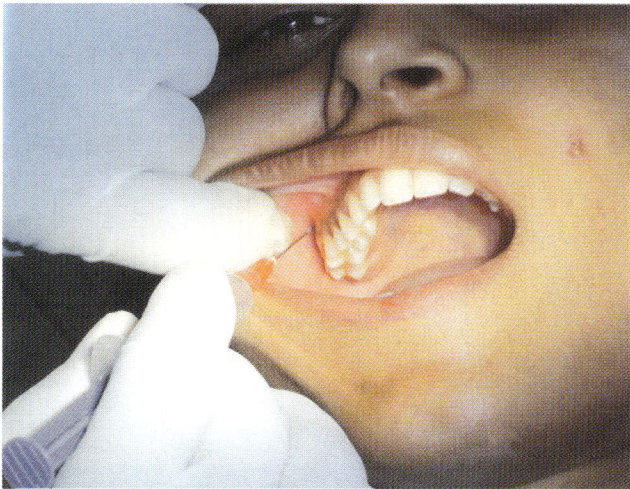

Fig. 7-4B: Position of the syringe and needle before insertion demonstrated in a patient. Note the 45° angulation of the syringe with the upper occlusal plane

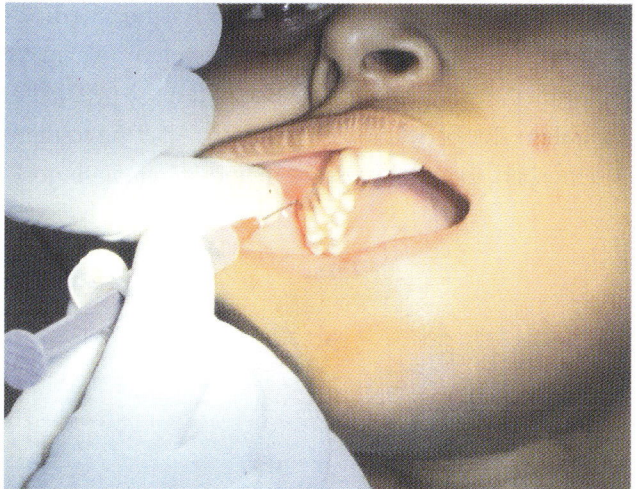

Fig. 7-5B: Position of the needle before depositing the solution for a superior alveolar nerve block. Note the angulation of the syringe to the occlusal plane is maintained at 45°

conform to the curvature of the tuberosity. The angulation of the syringe to the occlusal plane should be constantly maintained at 45° angulation (Figs 7-4B, 7-5A and B). The length of the needle inserted into the tisssues should not be more than ¾ of its length. Aspiration should be done before depositing the solution. If no blood is aspirated about 1cc of solution should be deposited and the needle is withdrawn. A separate injection is made near the mesiobucccal root of the 1st molar where few drops of solution is deposited. This is to anesthetize a branch of the middle superior alveolar nerve which supplies the mesiobuccal root.

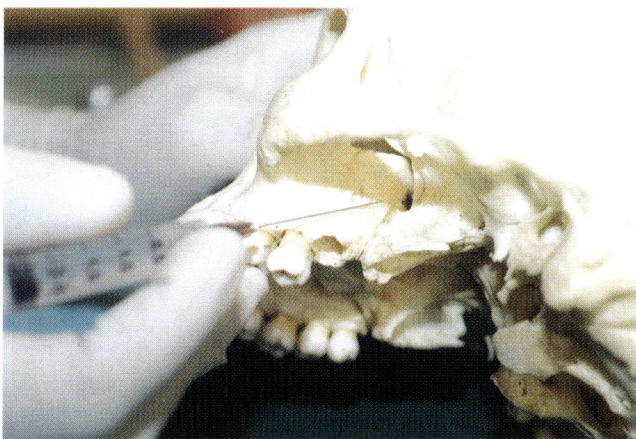

Fig. 7-5A: Position of the needle before depositing the solution, demonstrated on the tuberosity of the maxilla

The above injections anesthetize the mucous membrane covering the entire molar region on the buccal aspect, the periosteum, alveolar bone and the molar teeth.

INFRAORBITAL NERVE BLOCK

Infraorbital nerve block anesthesia is sometimes used when a minor surgery is to be carried out in the anterior maxillary region. This nerve block, anesthetizes the anterior and middle superior alveolar nerve. In the intraoral technique, the solution is deposited at the opening of the infraorbital foramen.

Injection Technique

The infraorbital foramen is palpated with the left index finger which is situated just below the infraorbital margin, the foramen is in line with the pupil of the eye, when the patient is looking straight forward. The intraoral landmark is the long axis of the 2nd premolar, which is in line with the infraorbital foramen (Figs 7-6A and B). The index finger of the left hand is kept in the infraorbital notch while retraction of the lip is done with the thumb. By retraction a clear view of the mucobuccal fold in the pre-molar region is visible. A disposable 2cc syringe with 1½ inch 26 gauge needle is loaded with the anesthetic solution. The needle is inserted in the periapical region of the 2nd premolar. The syringe is held parallel to the long axis of the 2nd molar tooth. As the needle is advanced towards the infraorbital foramen, it can be felt with the palpating index finger (Fig. 7-6C). After aspiration, 1cc of solution is deposited. After the solution is deposited, external pressure by the palpating finger is

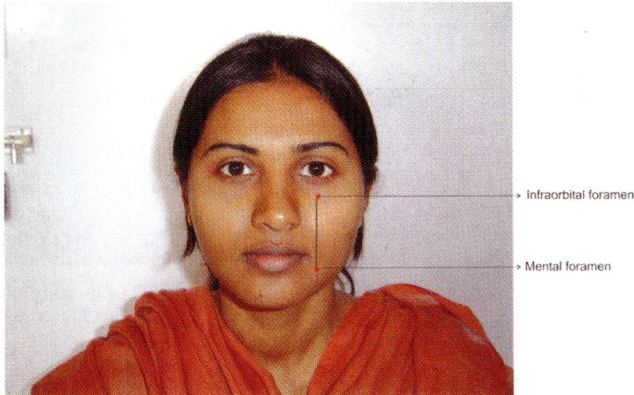

Fig. 7-6A: Orientation of infraorbital foramen on the face. A line drawn from the infraorbital foramen to the mental foramen. This is parallel to the long axis of 2nd premolar. This is also in line with the pupil of the eye when the patient is looking straight forward

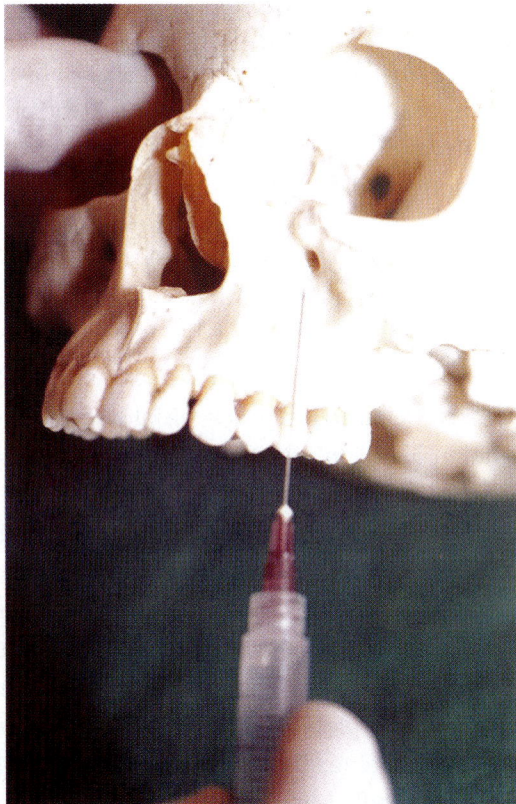

Fig. 7-6B: Position of the needle and syringe on the maxilla

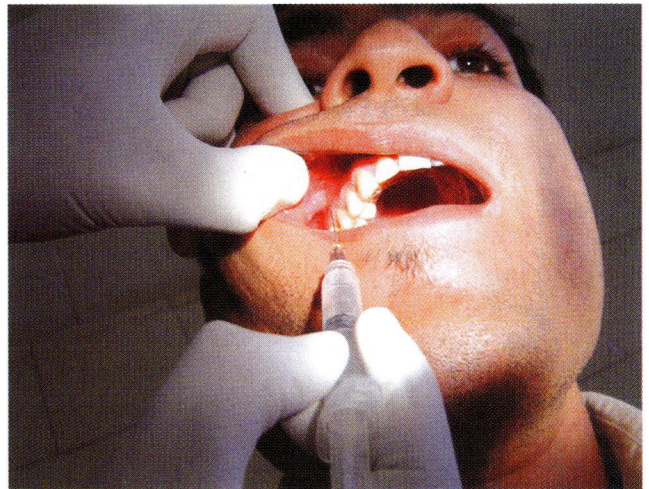

Fig. 7-6C: Position of the syringe and needle in a patient before giving the infraorbital block

applied, so as to force the solution through the foramen into the infraorbital canal. Many authors have advocated insertion of the needle by few cms into the canal, so that the solution is directly injected into the canal. Insertion of the needle into the canal can result in injury to the blood vessels or the nerve. Injury to the blood vessel can result in echymosis in the infraorbital region and the injury to the nerve can result in paresthesia. As the anesthesia of the region can be effectively obtained by simple infiltration technique the use of infraorbital block in dental practice is very rare.

PALATAL INJECTION

Mucous membrane of the hard palate is supplied by greater palatine and the nasopalatine nerve. Whenever extraction of the maxillary teeth is to be undertaken, anesthesia of the palatal mucous membrane becomes necessary. In these instances, local infiltration of the anesthetic solution below the palatal mucous membrane is made in the region corresponding to the tooth to be extracted. The insertion of the needle is usually done from the opposite side (Fig. 7-7A). After the insertion of the needle into the mucous membrane, the syringe is brought to an angulation of 30° to the buccal alveolar bone (Fig. 7-7B). This facilitates the easy flow of the solution while the solution is being deposited. Injection of 0.5 cc of anesthetic solution should result in anesthesia

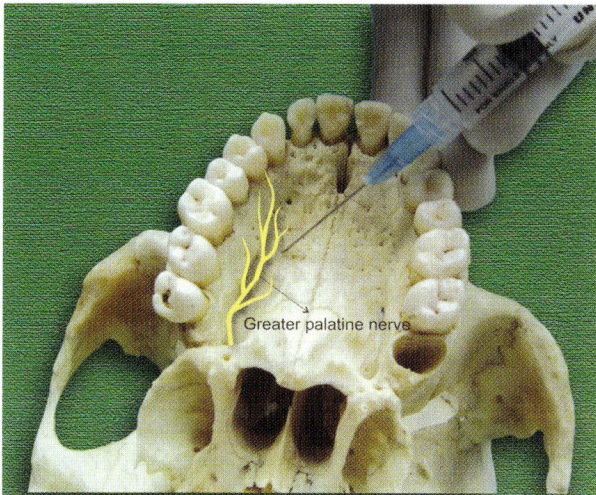

Fig. 7-7A: Position of the needle in the palatal region for anesthetizing greater palatine nerve branches

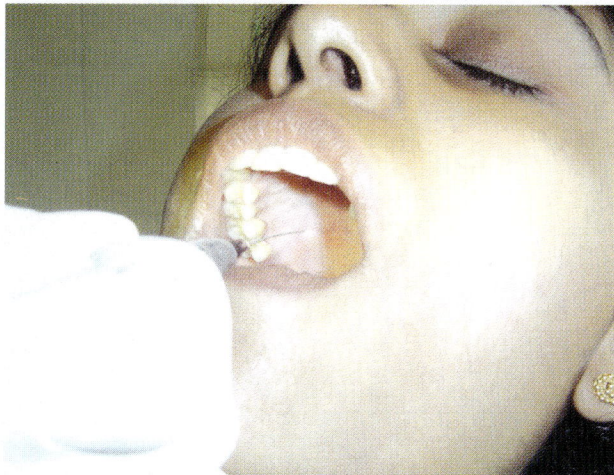

Fig. 7-7B: Position of the syringe and needle for a palatal injection. Note the paleness of the mucous membrane after depositing of the solution

of that local region. The deposition should be made slowly as a faster injection can result in pain during and also post-injection pain. In certain procedures, when wider area of palatal mucous membrane anesthesia is desired, nerve block of greater palatine nerve and nasopalatine nerve should be considered.

GREATER PALATINE NERVE BLOCK OR THE GREATER PALATINE CANAL INJECTION

The greater palatine nerve block anesthetizes the mucous membrane of the hard palate up to the premolar teeth. The injection is made from the opposite side with 1 inch

26 gauge needle. The point of insertion of the needle is between the 2nd and 3rd molar about 1 cm superior to the gingival margin. After insertion of the needle into the mucous membrane, the needle is kept at 30° angulation to the palatal alveolar bone and 0.5 ml of solution is slowly deposited near the foramen. There is no need to enter the canal as the deposition of the solution near the anterior palatine foramen should be sufficient to anesthetize the greater palatine nerve (Figs 7-8A to C).

NASOPALATINE NERVE BLOCK ANESTHESIA

This injection is made to obtain anesthesia of the palatal mucous membrane corresponding to the upper anterior

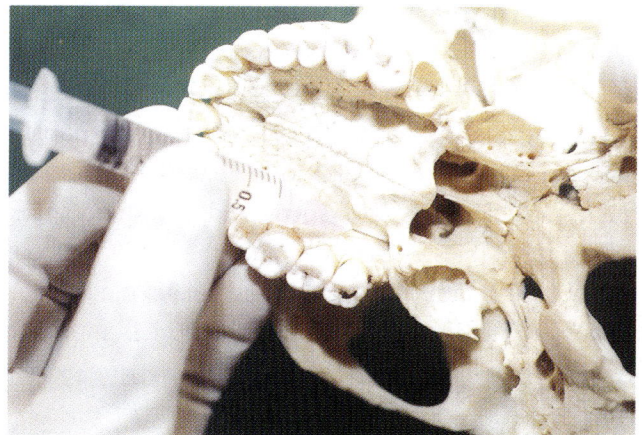

Fig. 7-8A: Needle in the greater palatine canal

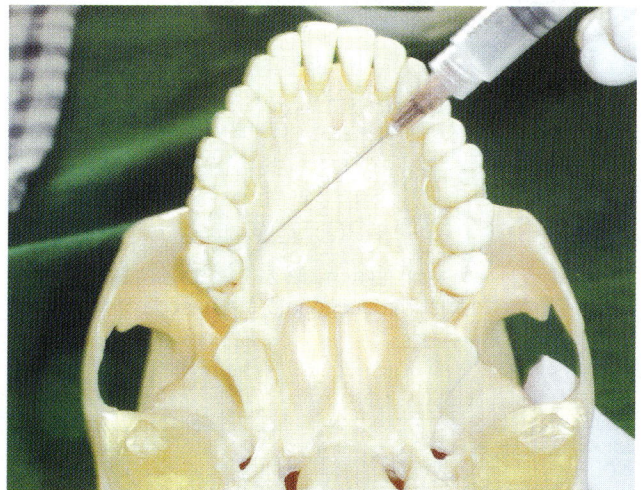

Fig. 7-8B: Place of deposition of the anesthetic solution

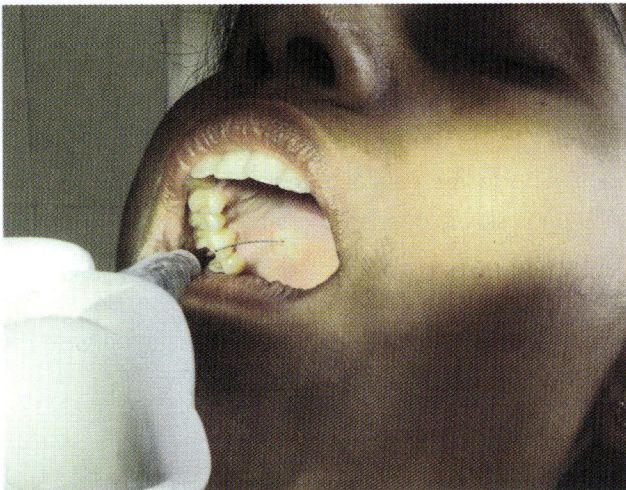

Fig. 7-8C: Injection for the greater palatine canal block anesthesia

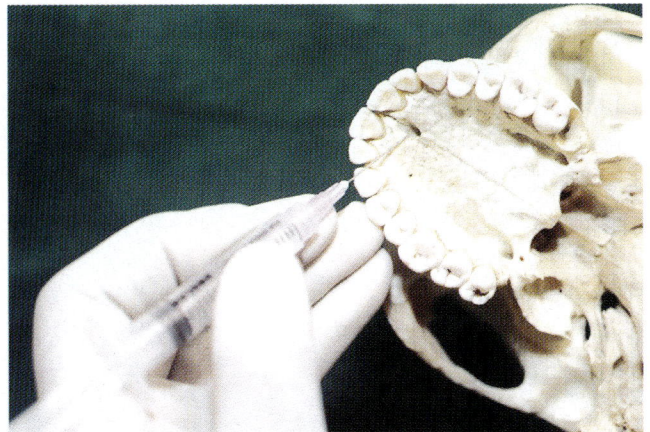

Fig. 7-9B: Place of deposition of solution near the opening of the incisive foramen

teeth. As the injection is very painful, anesthetic paste should be applied and massaged over the nasopalatine papilla before insertion of the needle. With a 1 inch 24 gauge needle, the insertion is made into the papilla, keeping the syringe parallel to the alveolar bone. Half ml of the solution is slowly deposited near the opening of the canal (Figs 7-9A to C). Since the palatal mucous membrane is firmly attached to the palate, the solution diffuses into the canal. This injection is made to

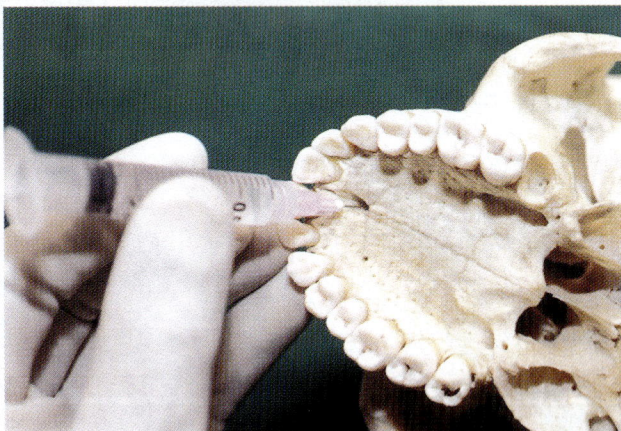

Fig. 7-9C: Injection and deposition of solution for nasopalatine nerve block

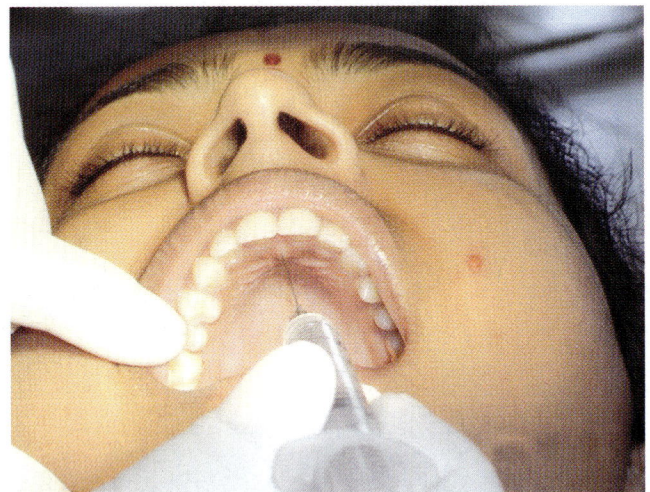

Fig. 7-9A: Needle introduced into the nasopalatine canal

supplement the infiltration made on the labial aspect before extraction of the anterior teeth. The palatal mucous membrane in the canine region is supplied by the branches of greater palatine nerve and also the nasopalatine nerve. Hence when a canine tooth is to be removed, to anesthetize the palatal mucous membrane, the injection should be made in the palatal region corresponding to the canine tooth.

8 Anesthesia in the Mandibular Region

Mandible is made up of thick cortical plates with abundant cancellous bone in between. The nature of cortical bone is dense (Fig. 8-1) except in the labial aspect in relation to lower anterior teeth. Due to this non-porous nature of the buccal cortical bone, local anesthesia in the mandibular region is achieved by block anesthesia. As the inferior alveolar nerve innervates all the teeth on one side of the jaw, it can be conveniently anesthetized by depositing local anesthetic solution in the region of the mandibular fossa just above the lingula of the mandibular foramen. The anesthesia of the supporting structures is achieved by lingual and long buccal nerve anesthesia. By anesthetizing the above three nerves, teeth on that particular side of the mandible extending from 2nd incisor to the 3rd molar, along with surrounding supporting structures are anesthetized. When only premolar teeth are required to be anesthetized a mental nerve block anesthesia can be adopted. Lower anterior teeth can be effectively anesthetized by infiltration technique as the bone covering the roots of these teeth are thin and porous in nature. In both the above injections when lingual mucous membrane anesthesia is desired a separate injection for the lingual nerve has to be given. Whenever extractions of lower central incisors are undertaken anesthetic solution has to be infiltrated on both sides of the midline on the labial and lingual aspect as there will crisscrossing of nerve fibers in the midline.

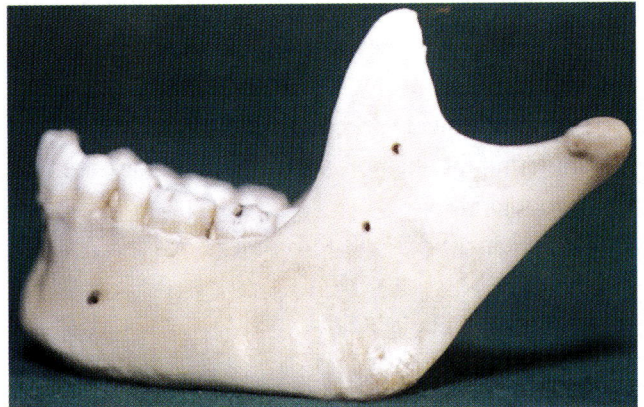

Fig. 8-1: Mandible—Note the non-porous nature of cortical alveolar bone

INFERIOR ALVEOLAR NERVE BLOCK

Before giving an inferior alveolar nerve block, the surgical anatomy of the area and certain anatomical landmarks should be considered. The mandibular foramen is situated on the medial surface of the ramus of the mandible (Fig. 8-3) in the pterygomandibular space. This space is bounded laterally by the inner surface of the mandible and medial pterygoid muscle on the medial side. Anteriorly it is limited by the superior constrictor muscle of the pharynx and the buccinator muscle. These two muscles are attached to the pterygomandibular raphe. Posteriorly it is bounded by the parotid gland (Fig. 8-2). The mandibular foramen is situated at the midpoint of the medial surface of the ramus of mandible. Its position from the anterior border of the ramus is approximately about 2.5 cm.

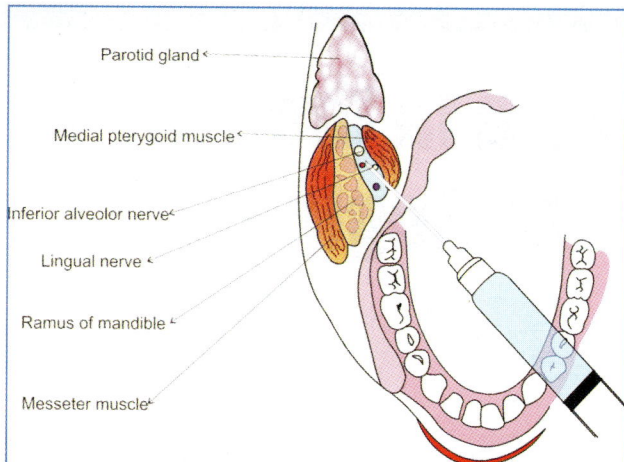

Fig. 8-2: Diagrammatic representation of the position of needle before depositing the anesthetic solution in the pterygomandibular space

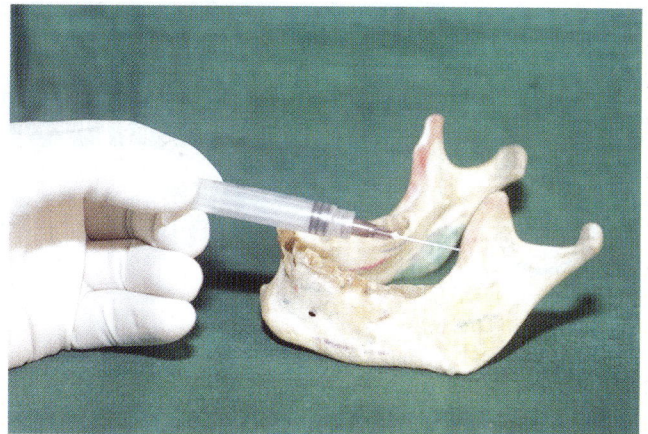

Fig. 8-4: Coronoid notch—This is the deepest point on the concavity of the anterior border of the ramus of mandible. Needle position just above the coronoid notch is shown

The anatomical landmarks which are helpful in administering the inferior alveolar nerve block are:

1. Coronoid notch
2. An imaginary plane 5 to 6 mm above the occlusal plane.
3. Pterygomandibular fold.
4. Inner oblique ridge.
5. External oblique ridge.

1. *Coronoid notch:* This is the deepest portion on the anterior border of the ramus of the mandible. This can be easily palpated by the index finger. This point represents the level at which the mandibular foramen

is present on the medial aspect of the ramus of the mandible. This landmark is more helpful in establishing the level at which the foramen is present in edentulous patients (Fig. 8.4).

2. *An imaginary plane 5 to 6 mm above the occlusal plane (Fig. 8-5):*
   This plane is at the level of coronoid notch and hence corresponds to the mandibular foramen on the medial aspect of the ramus. In dentulous patients, it is convenient to imagine this plane and sometimes the location of the mandibular foramen can be easily established without palpating the coronoid notch.

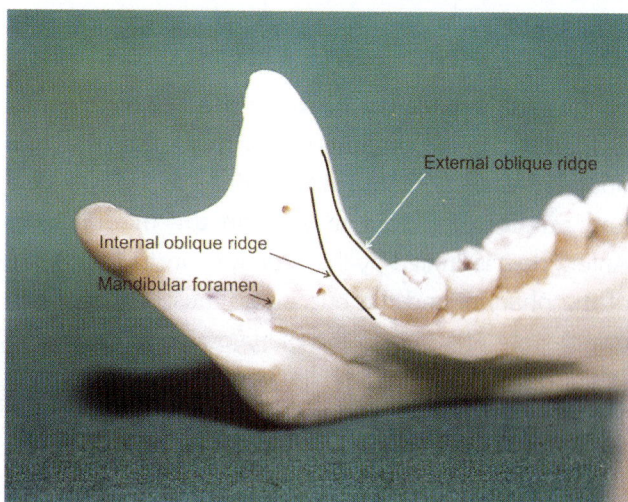

Fig. 8-3: Medial surface of the mandible showing the position of mandibular foramen in relation to coronoid notch and inner oblique ridge

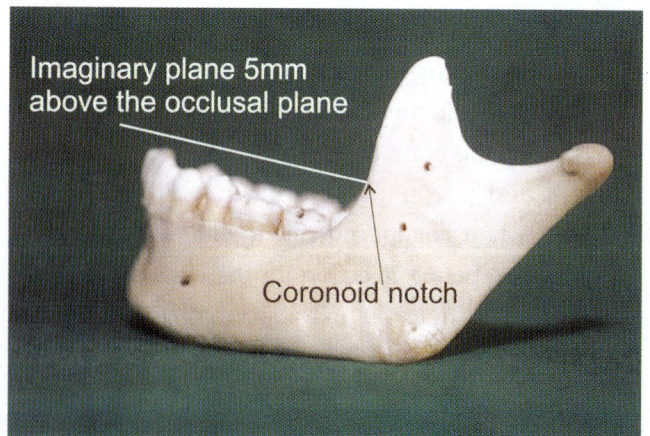

Fig. 8-5: The imaginary plane 5 to 6 mm above the occlusal plane. This plane is at the same level of the coronoid notch and the mandibular foramen

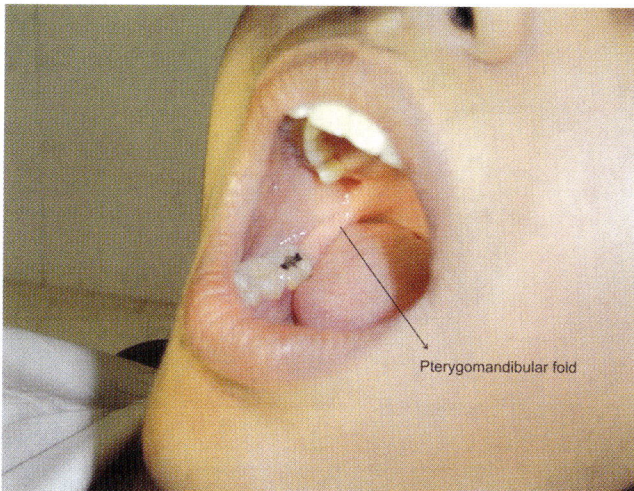

Fig. 8-6: Pterygomandibular fold

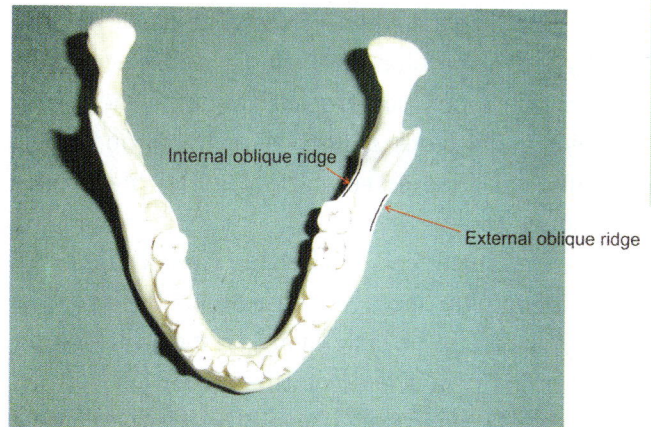

Fig. 8-7: External and internal oblique ridge

3. *Pterygomandibular fold (Fig. 8-6):* This is a mucosal fold which is prominently seen at the retromandibular area when the patient opens the mouth wide open. This fold is formed by the pterygomandibular raphe covered by the mucous membrane. The pterygomandibular raphe extends from the pterygoid hamulus and the posterior end of the mylohyoid ridge on the lingular aspect, immediately adjacent to the 3rd molar tooth. The ligament gives attachment on its anterior region to the buccinator muscle, and on its posterior aspect to the anterior constrictor muscle of the pharynx. The pterygomandibular fold is an important landmark in locating the point of insertion of the needle for the inferior alveolar nerve block anesthesia.

4. *Inner oblique ridge:* This ridge is palpable just lateral to the pterygomandibular fold. The palpation of the landmark establishes the position of the ridge (Figs 8-3 and 8-7). The point of needle insertion is situated between the pterygomandibular fold and the inner oblique ridge. Usually the point of needle insertion is about 3 to 5 mm lateral to the pterygomandibular fold. Inserting the needle too far laterally will lead into the retromolar triangle. Again insertion of the needle too far medially can lead beyond the mandibular foramen.

5. *External oblique ridge:* The external oblique ridge extends upwards and merges with the anterior border of the ramus of mandible (Figs 8-3 and 8-7). Palpation of this border gives an idea about the angulation of the ramus to the body of the mandible. If the deflection of the ramus is more, the needle may have to be inserted a little more than what is normal.

Technique of Injection

When mandibular molar teeth are to be extracted, an inferior alveolar nerve block is preferred. The inferior alveolar nerve block although indicates blocking of the inferior alveolar nerve; the term is generally referred to anesthetizing the inferior alveolar nerve, lingual nerve and long buccal nerve. This block sometimes is referred to as mandibular block.

The inferior alveolar nerve block can be administered by two methods. In the first method, the long buccal nerve is anesthetized first at the retromolar triangle and secondly the lingual nerve and lastly the inferior alveolar nerve. Since the approach to the inferior alveolar nerve is indirect, the technique is termed as Indirect technique. In the second method which is termed as direct, visual or classic technique, the inferior alveolar nerve at the mandibular fossa is approached directly in the first instant. When the needle is being withdrawn, the lingual and long buccal nerves are anesthetized. For beginners it is advisable to practise the indirect method a few times before practising the direct method. The classic method of alveolar nerve block is a simple, easier and most popular technique. Success or effectiveness of the inferior alveolar nerve block entirely depends upon understanding the landmarks and mastering the proper technique.

It is convenient and comfortable if one can practise administering the injection with both hands. Injections can be given conveniently sitting on the right side for anesthetizing right sided teeth (Fig. 8-8A) and on the left side for left sided teeth (Fig. 8-8B). This gives a clear view of the injection area and will avoid unnecessary leaning on the patient's body while administering anesthesia on the opposite site of the jaw. Techniques advocated in many textbooks do recommend a right front position for right-handed operators. At a later stage the author feels that this can be practised as is convenient to each individual.

Classic Technique

The patient is comfortably seated in a semi-reclining position. The area of injection should be clearly visible under well directed light. The landmarks are palpated by the palpating finger. The pulp of the index finger is placed in the retromolar triangle with finger kept parallel to the buccal surfaces of teeth and the occlusal level. The mid point of the nail on the forefinger represents

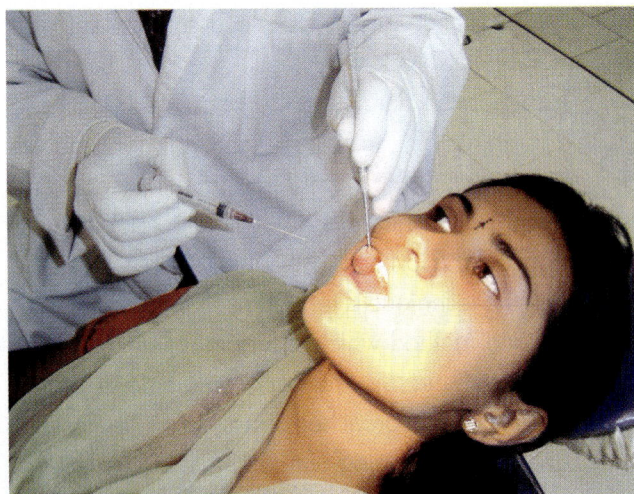

Fig. 8-8B: Position of the operator on the left side of the patient. Syringe is held in left hand

the point of insertion of the needle. This also corresponds to the coronoid notch and an imaginary plane 5 to 6 mm above the occlusal plane. Alternatively the point can be marked by a marker on the mucous membrane and the finger can be retracted or withdrawn (Fig. 8-9).

The cheek can be retracted by a finger or a mouth mirror. This gives a clear view of the retromolar area and the pterygomandibular fold (Fig. 8-10). A 2 cc syringe with 1½ inch 26 gauge needle, loaded with the anesthetic solution is positioned 5 to 6 mm above the occlusal plane

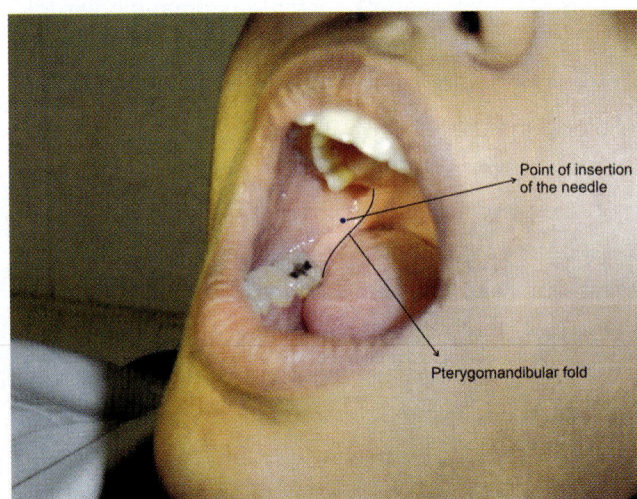

Fig. 8-8A: Position of the operator on the right side of the patient. Syringe is held in right hand

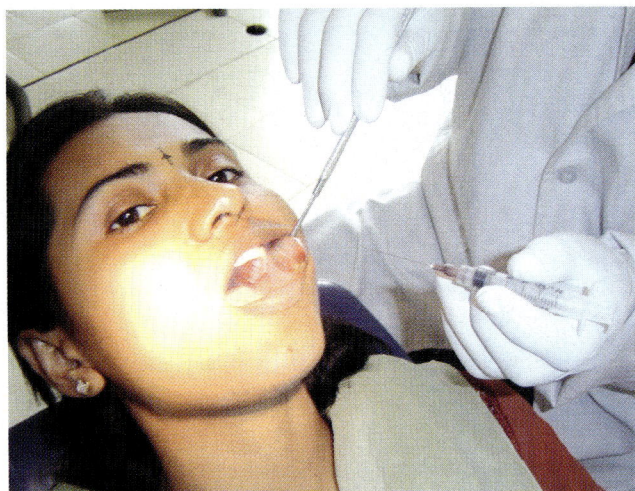

Point of insertion of the needle

Pterygomandibular fold

Fig. 8-9: Shows the point of insertion of the needle lateral to the pterygomandibular fold and medial to the internal oblique ridge. This point can be marked by a marking pen

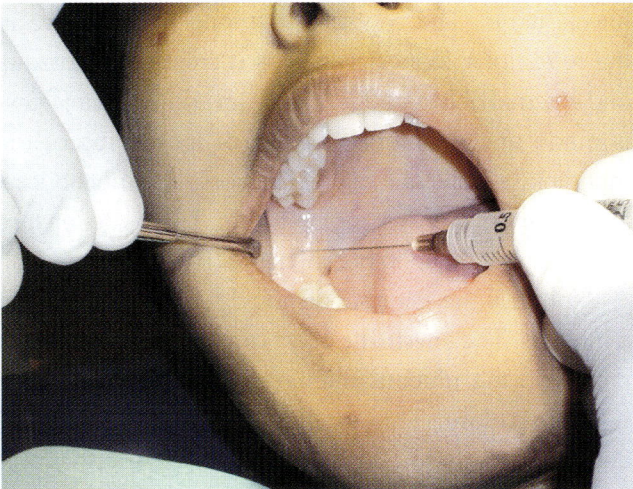

Fig. 8-10: Cheek retraction is being done by a mouth mirror to give a clear view of the retromolar area

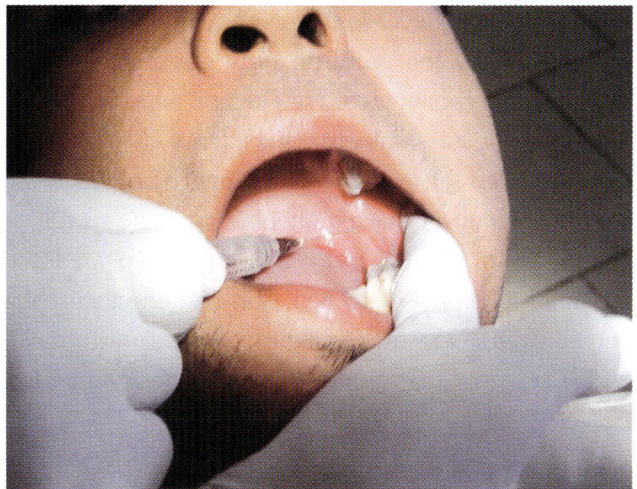

Fig. 8-11B: Position of the right index finger and the syringe held in the right hand for a left inferior alveolar nerve block. Here the hands are kept in scissors form

from the opposite pre-molar area (Figs 8-11A and B). The needle is inserted into the mucous membrane corresponding to midpoint of the nail of forefinger or at the point of marking. The needle is inserted to a depth of 2 to 2.5 cm, at which stage the needle should encounter the bone (Fig. 8-11C). In some patients due to the deflexion of the ramus, the depth of insertion may be 2 to 3 mm more than normal. If the needle does not make contact with bone even after the needle is inserted to a depth of 2.5 cm, then it is better to recheck the position of the syringe and the point of insertion of

the needle. Once the needle makes contact with the bone, the syringe should be withdrawan for 1 to 2 mm. Aspiration of the syringe should be done and 1.5 ml of solution should be slowly deposited. It is important that the syringe should be kept parallel to the occlusal plane throughout the proceedure. Some patients do not tolerate the presence of the syringe in the oral cavity and tend to push the syringe with the tongue. This might change the angulation of the syringe and the tip of the needle may be directed downwards. This results in the solution being deposited below the mandibular fossa. To prevent this, the tongue should be held laterally with a mouth mirror. Alternatively, the needle insertion is

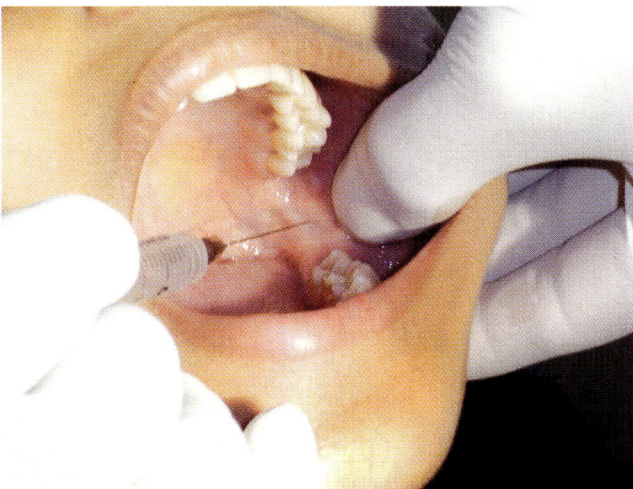

Fig. 8-11A: Position of thumb, syringe and needle for a left inferior alveolar nerve block

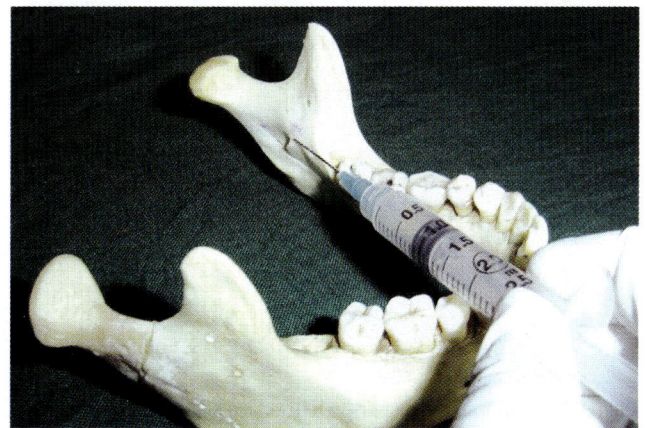

Fig. 8-11C: Position of the syringe and needle for the direct technique—demonstrated on the mandible

done at a higher level so that even when the syringe is slightly tilted, the solution gets deposited at the mandibular foramen area. The solution deposited at the mandibular fossa anesthetizes the inferior alveolar nerve before it enters the mandibular foramen. After depositing 1.5 ml solution at the mandibular fossa the needle is withdrawn for about 1 inch. Aspiration is repeated and 0.5 ml of solution is deposited. This is to anesthetize the lingual nerve. Now the needle is completely withdrawn and a separate injection is made for the long buccal nerve.

Alternatively after depositing the anesthetic solution at the mandibular foramen and the needle having been withdrawn for 1 inch, the syringe is swung to the same side keeping it parallel to the occlusal plane. Aspiration is repeated and 0.5 ml of solution is deposited. This will anesthetize the lingual nerve which runs close to the bone near the 3rd molar tooth. By swinging the syringe to the same side, the syringe can be held more steadily as the needle stays in close contact with inner oblique ridge and the patient feels more comfortable with the syringe on the buccal side than across the arch (Fig. 8-12).

As the syringe is being withdrawn, 0.2 cc of the solution is deposited, which should anesthetize the long buccal nerve. The course of the long buccal nerve in the retromolar triangle varies as it crosses the internal and external oblique ridge. Hence an additional injection is made at the anterior border of the ramus of the mandible, slightly at a higher level or at the mucobuccal fold near to the 3rd molar tooth. This is to ensure anesthesia of the long buccal nerve (Figs 8-13A and B).

Normally the anesthesia should take its effect within 5 minutes. The anesthetic effect can be tested by a sharp probe on the mucous membrane between the lower two premolars. This would give an indication of anesthesia of the inferior alveolar nerve. Anesthesia of the long buccal nerve can be tested on the mucous membrane in the molar region.

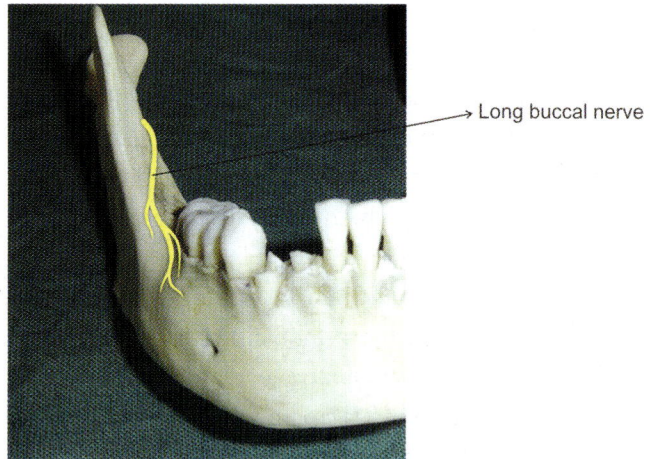

Fig. 8-13A: Course of the long buccal nerve in relation to inner and external oblique ridge

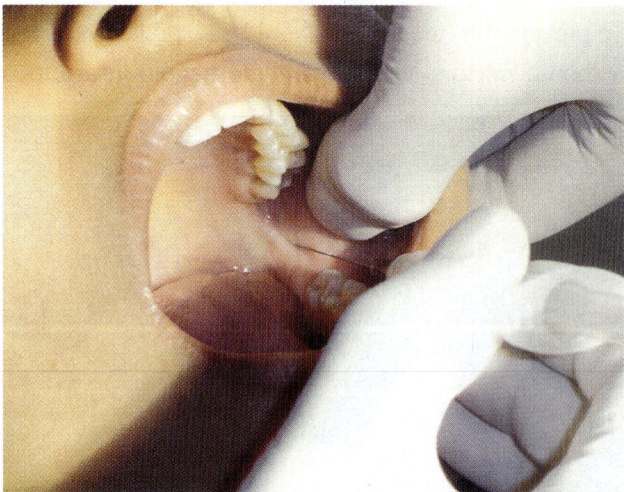

Fig. 8-12: Swinging the syringe to the same side. This is carried out after depositing the solution for the inferior alveolar nerve. Patient will feel more comfortable with the syringe on the side of the cheek

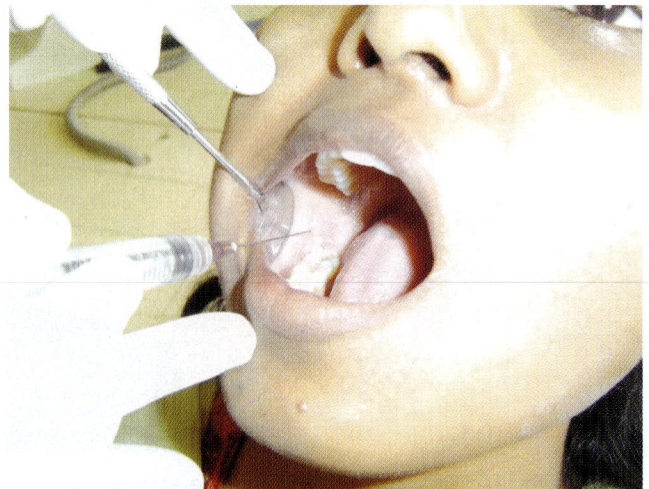

Fig. 8-13B: Injection for the long buccal nerve

Indirect Techniques of Inferior Alveolar Nerve Block

In this technique, same landmarks as described in the direct technique are considered and palpated. The needle insertion is at the level of coronoid notch and just medial to the inner oblique ridge of mandible. The needle is inserted at the designated point while the syringe is held at the lower premolars on the opposite side. After inserting the needle to a depth of 2 mm a few drops of anesthetic solution is deposited to anesthetize the long buccal nerve. The needle is further advanced to a depth of 1 cm and 0.5 ml of solution is deposited after aspiration. This should anesthetize the lingual nerve. Now the needle is inserted to a further depth of 1.5 cm. At this stage the needle should make contact with the bone at the mandibular foramen. The needle is withdrawn for 1 or 2 mm, aspiration is done and 1.5 ml of anesthetic solution is deposited to anesthetize the inferior alveolar nerve. After withdrawing the needle a separate injection for the long buccal nerve is made.

Alternatively the syringe is held parallel to the buccal surfaces of teeth on the same side. After insertion of the needle at the designated point to a depth of 2mm, a few drops of anesthetic solution is deposited in this position, which should anesthetize the long buccal nerve. The needle is further inserted to an additional depth of 1cm, avoiding the inner oblique ridge. In this position, 0.5 ml of solution is deposited to anesthetize the lingual nerve. Now the syringe is swung to the opposite side to the pre-molar region. The needle is further inserted where the bone is encountered. The syringe is withdrawn for 1 to 2 mm. Aspiration is done before depositing 1.5 ml of the anesthetic solution at the mandibular fossa to anesthetize the inferior alveolar nerve. The position of the syringe should be kept parallel to the occlusal plane during the process of injection.

Alternative Techniques for Inferior Alveolar Nerve Block Anesthesia

Clark and Holmes (1959) explained a technique for anesthetizing the inferior alveolar nerve which is similar to the indirect technique except that the needle insertion is 1.5 cm above the occlusal plane (Fig. 8-14). In this technique the anesthetic solution is deposited in the mandibular fossa at a little higher level to the mandibular foramen. This enables anesthesia of any small branches arising from inferior alveolar nerve, before it enters the mandibular foramen.

Angelo Sargenti (1966) explained a technique similar to the direct technique. The anesthetic solution is deposited at a higher level to the mandibular foramen. In this technique the syringe is placed in contact with occlusal surface of upper premolars of the opposite side.

In patients who have difficulty in opening the mouth, the intraoral technique for inferior alveolar nerve block described by *Sundar.J.Vazirani (1960)* can be adopted. In this technique, the cheek is fully retracted and the needle insertion is immediately medial to the anterior border of the ramus of mandible. The syringe is placed parallel to the gingiva of the maxillary teeth (Fig. 8-15). The needle is inserted to a depth of 1.5 cms. The syringe is aspirated and the anesthetic solution deposited. As the deposition of the solution is slightly away from the inner surface of the ramus of mandible, it is

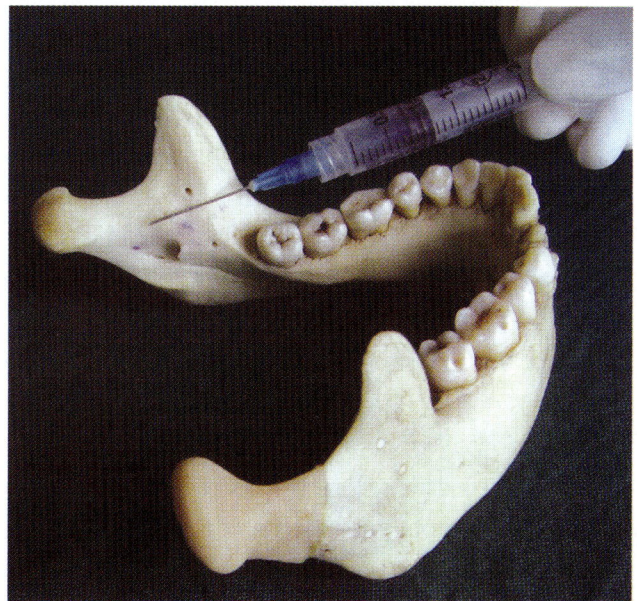

Fig. 8-14: Position of the needle to show the place of deposition of anesthetic solution in Clark and Holmes technique of inferior alveolar nerve block

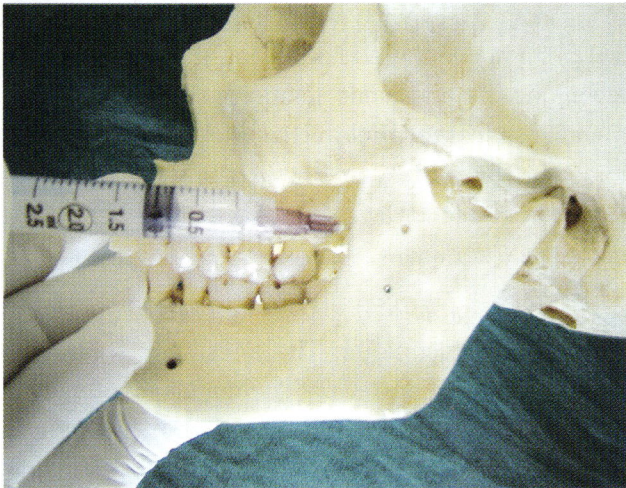

Fig. 8-15: Position of needle and syringe for an intraoral inferior alveolar nerve block by Sunder Vazirani technique

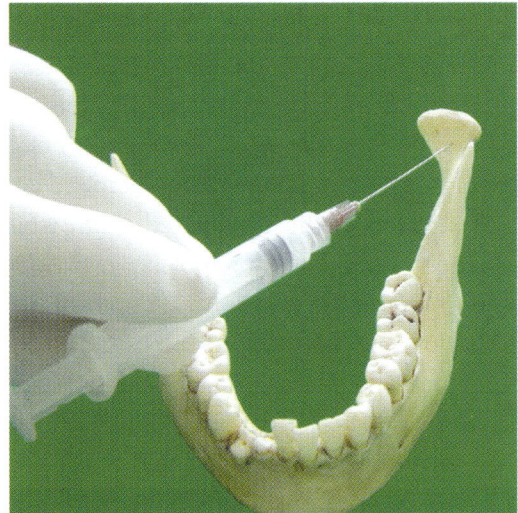

Fig. 8-16A: Point of deposition of anesthetic solution in a Gow-Gates technique

recommended to use 2.5 ml or 3 ml of anesthetic solution. The long buccal nerve can be anesthetized by a separate injection, by depositing a few drops of the solution on the external oblique ridge near the 3rd molar tooth.

Gow-Gates Technique

In this technique, the anesthetic solution is deposited near the anterior surface of the head of the condyle (Fig. 8-16A). This procedure is carried out by an intraoral approach with extraoral landmarks for correct positioning of the needle. Extraoral landmark is a line drawn from the corner of the mouth to the intratragic notch (Fig. 8-16B). The patient is asked to open the mouth wide, so that the condyle is placed in the forward position. Intraorally the anterior border of the ramus of the mandible is palpated and the finger is moved upwards to feel for the tendon of temporalis muscle. The needle insertion is done in the mucous membrane, just medial to the tendon of temporalis muscle. The syringe is kept parallel to the extra-oral line (Fig. 8-16C). The insertion of the needle is from the opposite side (Fig. 8-16D) and the depth of insertion should not exceed 25 mm. When the anterior surface of the head condyle is felt by the needle, the syringe is withdrawn for 1 mm or 2 mm and

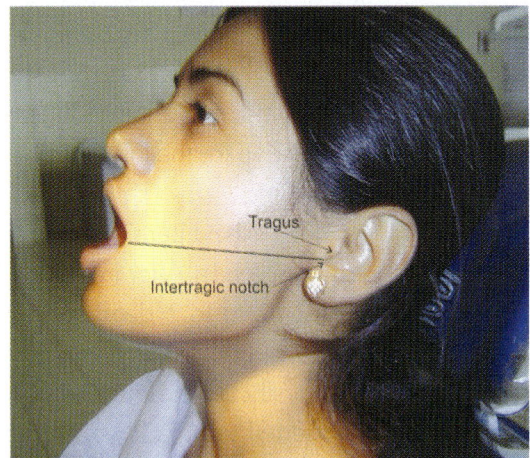

Fig. 8-16B: External surface markings for Gow-Gates technique of mandibular nerve block

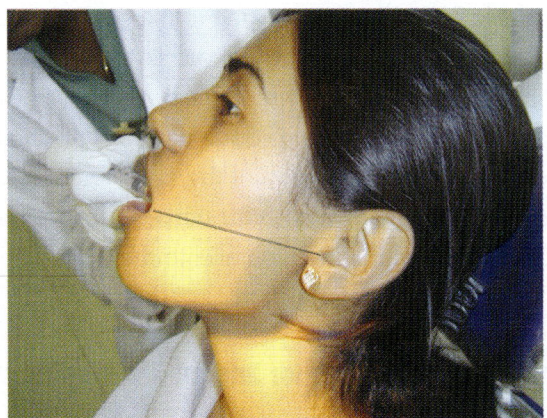

Fig. 8-16C: Position of syringe in relation to external markings

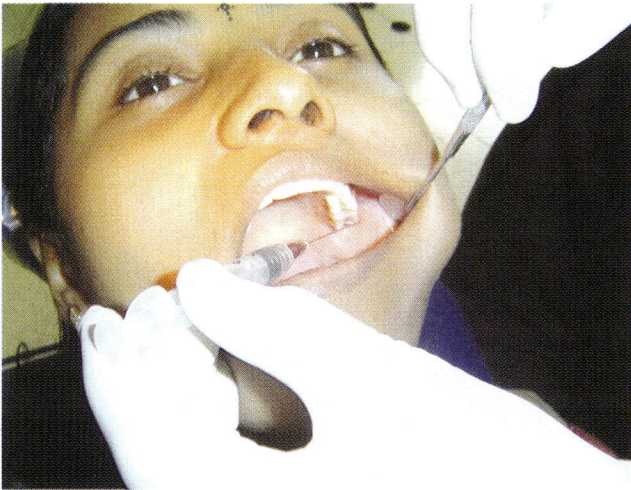

Fig. 8-16D: Point of needle insertion in Gow-Gates mandibular nerve block

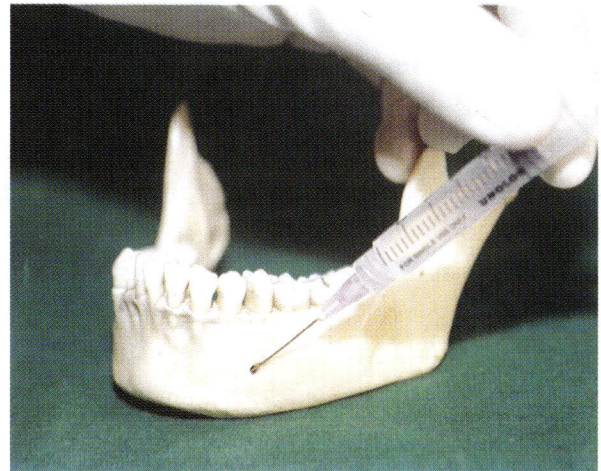

Fig. 8-17A: Needle inserted into mental foramen to show the direction of opening

the solution is deposited. This will anesthetize the entire mandibular nerve.

MENTAL NERVE BLOCK ANESTHESIA

Mental nerve is a branch of inferior alveolar nerve and it emerges from the mental foramen which is situated in between the two premolar teeth. Although this block of anesthesia is termed as mental nerve block it is administered to anesthetize the incisive nerve and the branch supplying the 1st premolar. To achieve anesthesia of lower anterior teeth and the 1st premolar the anesthetic solution has to diffuse through the mental foramen. This block of anesthesia infact should be termed as incisive nerve block although the injection also anesthetizes the mental nerve.

Technique: The cheek is retracted to have a clear view of the mucobuccal fold in the premolar region. The direction of approach should be from posterio superior direction (Figs 8-17A to C) as the mental foramen opens posterio superiorly. A two ml syringe with 24 gauge 1-inch needle loaded with 1.5 ml of anesthetic solution is used. The needle insertion should be at the periapical region of 2nd premolar and is directed forwards to a

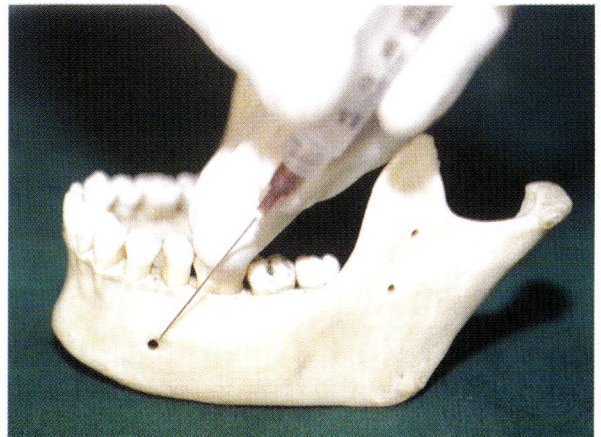

Fig. 8-17B: Place of deposition of anesthetic solution

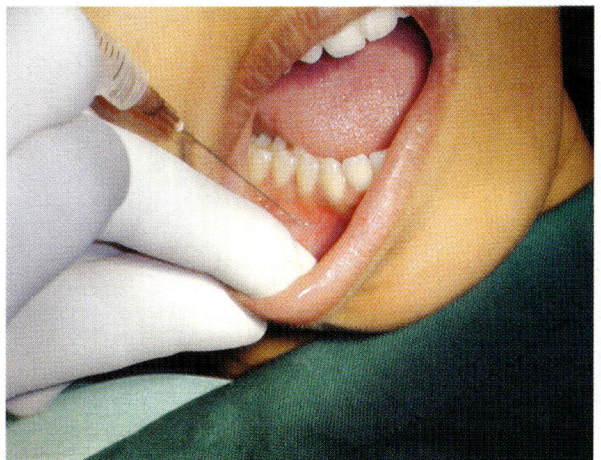

Fig. 8-17C: Mental nerve block being demonstrated in a patient

depth of 1 cm close to the bone. The needle is held at 20° angulation to the buccal bone. Aspiration is done before depositing 1 ml of solution. The needle is withdrawn and light external massaging is done in the area to facilitate flow of solution into the canal through the mental foramen.

By this injection the anterior teeth, 1st premolar, alveolar bone, periosteum, buccal mucous membrane in that region and the lower lip on that side is anesthetized. When extraction of the anterior teeth and the 1st premolar is to be undertaken, it becomes necessary to anesthetize the lingual mucous membrane as this is supplied by lingual nerve. The lingual nerve is anesthetized by injecting 0.5 cc of solution in the lingual mucous membrane in relation to that particular tooth. Whenever the central incisor is to be extracted a few drops of solution has to be injected in the periapical region of the opposite central incisor. This is to anesthetize the nerve fibers from the opposite side (Figs 8-18B and C).

INFILTRATION TECHNIQUES IN MANDIBULAR REGION

The bone covering the lower incisors are quite thin and porous in nature (Fig. 8-18A). To anesthetize the incisor teeth infiltration anesthesia can be utilized as the solution

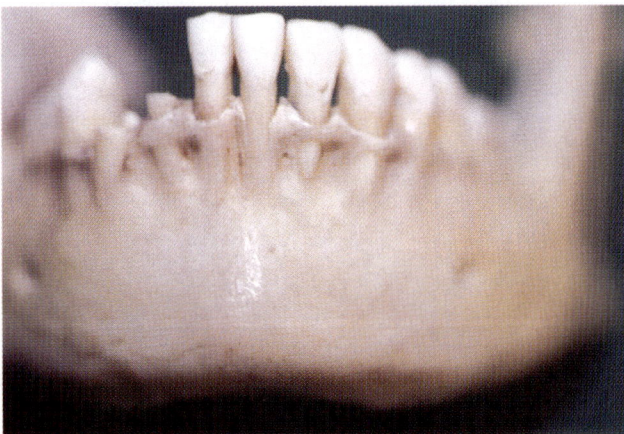

Fig. 8.18B

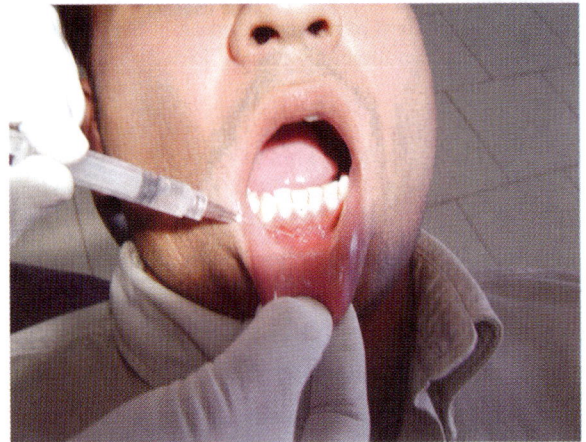

Figs 8-18B and C: Infiltration anesthesia of the lower right central incisor. Here the solution has to be infiltrated apart from at the periapical region of the particular tooth into the area beyond the midline

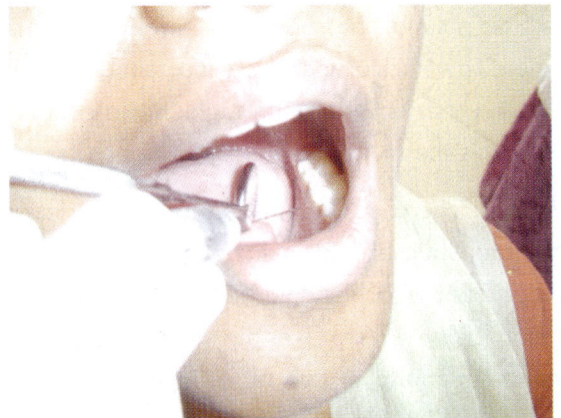

Fig. 8-18A: Anterior region of the mandible shows thinness of the labial bone and the porous nature of alveolar bone

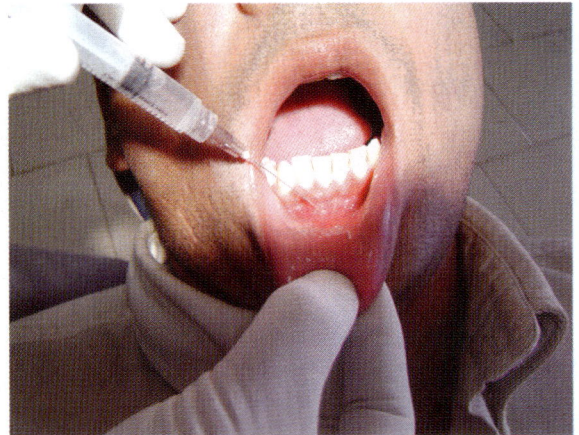

Fig. 8-19: Lingual nerve block anesthesia

easily diffuses through the labial plate of bone. Apart from this, infiltration cannot be used to anesthetize any other teeth in the mandible.

Lingual nerve has to be anesthetized by a separate injection to anesthetize the lingual mucous membrane. The injection can be made below the mucous membrane in the region of 2nd molar tooth close to the bone (Fig. 8-19). Half cc of anesthetic solution should be sufficient to anesthetize the lingual nerve on that side.

<table>
<tr><td>9</td><td># Extraoral Local Anesthesia Techniques</td></tr>
</table>

Extraoral anesthesia techniques can be adopted for the maxillary nerve, mandibular nerve, infraorbital nerve and the inferior alveolar nerve. In these techniques, although certain external landmarks are used (Fig. 9-1A) it should be kept in mind that, the progress of the needle is in a highly vascular area. This may result in internal bleeding and also injure nerve tissue and muscle tissue. In dental practice application of extraoral block are very rare and not very essential. Local anesthesia may be conveniently achieved without any complication by intraoral procedures.

EXTRAORAL MAXILLARY NERVE BLOCK

In this block the solution is deposited in the pterygopalatine fossa to anesthetize the maxillary nerve before it divides into various branches. The point of insertion of the needle is in the center of the depression below the lower border of zygomatic arch in front of the eminence of the condylar fossa (Fig. 9-1B). A 4 inch 22 gauge needle attached to a luer-loc syringe is used in this technique. Depth of insertion is 2 inches and is marked on the needle with a rubber stopper. The needle is inserted at the marked spot with syringe held perpendicular to the skin surface. The needle insertion is done up to the rubber stopper at which depth it should make contact with pterygoid plate. Now the needle is withdrawn for 1 to 1½ inch and inserted in a superior and anterior direction (Fig. 9-1C). Once the maximum depth is reached aspiration is done and 2 ml of anesthetic solution is deposited.

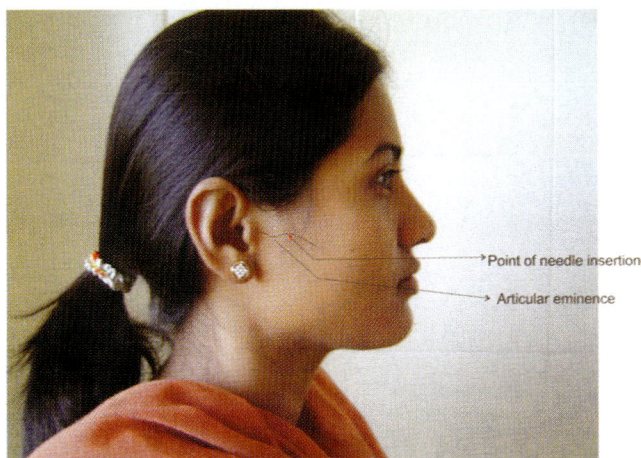

Fig. 9-1A: External markings for extraoral block anesthesia for both mandibular and maxillary nerve

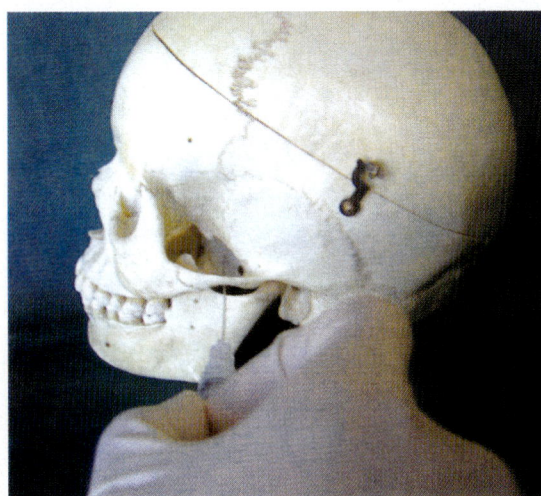

Fig. 9-1B: Initial position of needle for both mandibular nerve and maxillary nerve anesthesia by extraoral approach demonstrated on the skull

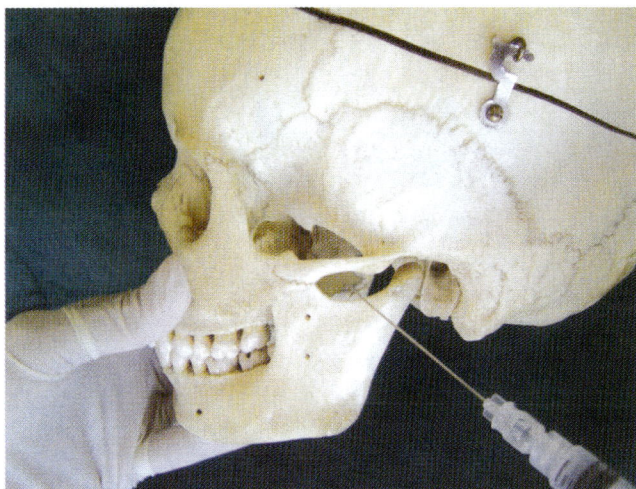

Fig. 9-1C: Position of needle for the maxillary nerve anesthesia

EXTRAORAL MANDIBULAR NERVE BLOCK

The landmarks for this block are similar to the maxillary nerve block. The anesthetic solution in this technique is deposited in the region of foramen ovale. In this method once the needle touches the pterygoid plate it is withdrawn for 1 inch and redirected posterior to the lateral pterygoid plate (Fig. 9-1D) to a further distance of 4 mm. At this stage aspiration is done and the anesthetic solution is deposited. This should anesthetize the entire mandibular nerve.

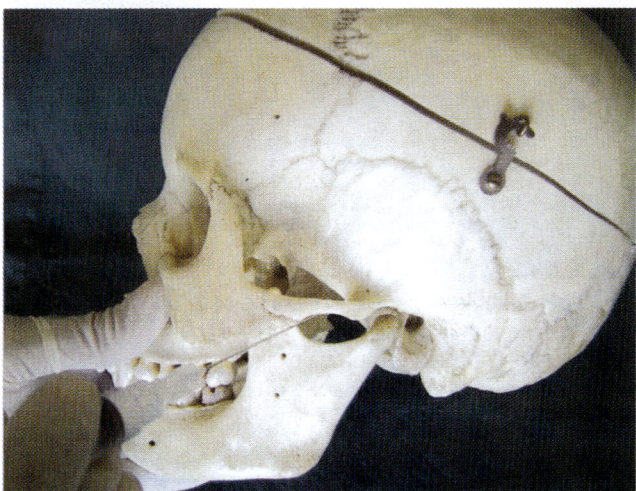

Fig. 9-1D: Position of needle for the mandibular nerve anesthesia

EXTRAORAL INFRAORBITAL NERVE BLOCK

The infraorbital foramen can be easily palpated just below the infraorbital ridge (Fig. 9-2A). The finger while palpating, dips into the hollow of the fossa below the foramen. The index finger is placed in this region. The needle insertion is 1 cm below the foramen. The syringe is kept at 40° angulation. After inserting the needle up to the bone aspiration is done and 0.5 ml of solution is deposited. After 1 minute the needle is advanced superiorly and slow progress is made for 2 or 3 mm into the canal through the opening (Fig. 9-2B). Slow deposition of the solution is done with the index finger firmly placed in the area.

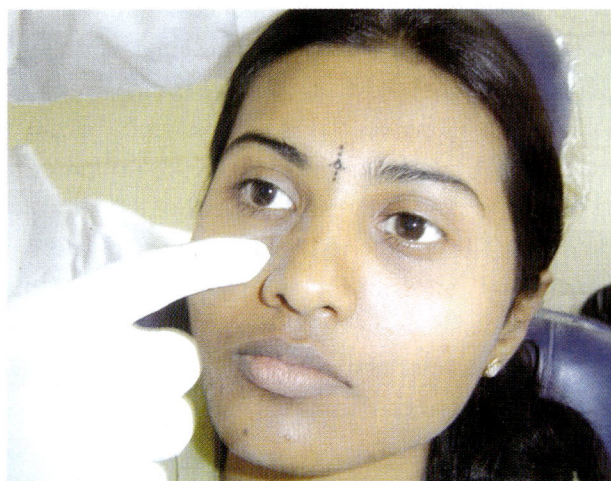

Fig. 9-2A: Palpation of the infraorbital foramen and fossa

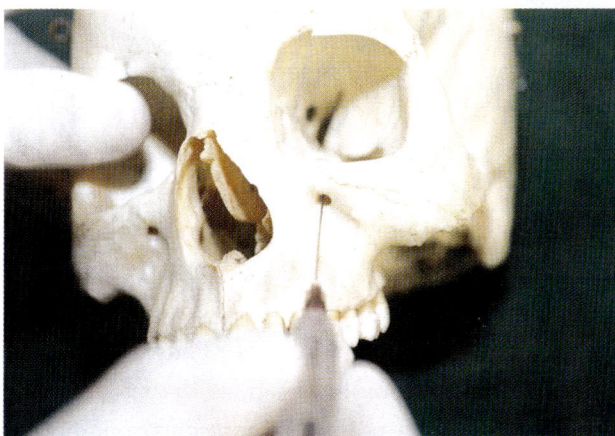

Fig. 9-2B: Location and direction of the canal shown by introducing the needle through infraorbital foramen

INFERIOR ALVEOLAR NERVE BLOCK BY EXTERNAL APPROACH

This technique was first explained by professor Kurt Thoma and can be used to anesthetize the inferior alveolar nerve with an extra-oral approach. This approach is useful in patients with severe trismus or ankylosis of the TMJ. The anterior border of the masseter is marked at the lower border of mandible. This can be easily palpated when the patient clenches his teeth. From this point, a straight line is drawn to the tragus of the ear. Midpoint of this line is marked. This midpoint represents the mandibular foramen on the inner surface of the ramus of mandible. From this point, a vertical line parallel to the ramus of the mandible is drawn up to the lower border of mandible. The length from the midpoint to lower border of mandible is measured and marked on the long needle by a sterile rubber stopper. The needle is inserted from below the lower border of the mandible close to the inner surface of the ramus of mandible. The needle is inserted up to the rubber stopper. Aspiration of the syringe is done and the anesthetic solution is deposited. This should anesthetize the inferior alveolar nerve. The lingual nerve and the long buccal nerve can be anesthetized by an intraoral buccal approach.

Alternatively to locate the mandibular foramen the following landmarks can be considered. The lower border and posterior border of the mandible are marked. The point of attachment of masseter muscle anteriorly (point A) is marked as in case of previous technique. Angle of the mandible is marked (point E) A line from the corner of mouth to the attachment of lobe of the ear is made. This should correspond to the imaginary plane 5 to 6 mm above the occlusal plane. This will also correspond to the coronoid notch and the mandibular foramen. A line parallel to posterior border of ramus of mandible from point B (midpoint of A E) is drawn upto the horizontal line. The point 'C' represents mandibular foramen (Fig. 9-3A). The distance is measured and marked on the needle by a rubber stopper (Fig. 9-3B). The point of insertion of the needle is at point 'D' below

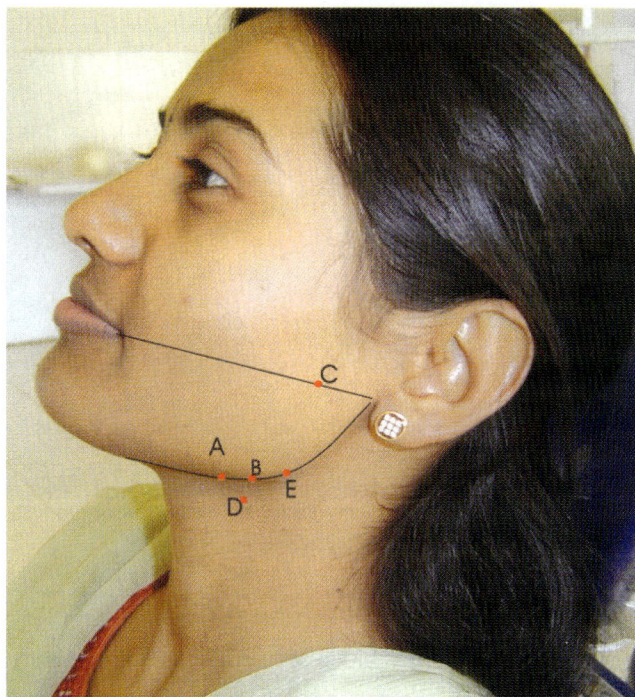

Fig. 9-3A: Extraoral markings for the alternate technique for inferior alveolar nerve block anesthesia through external approach

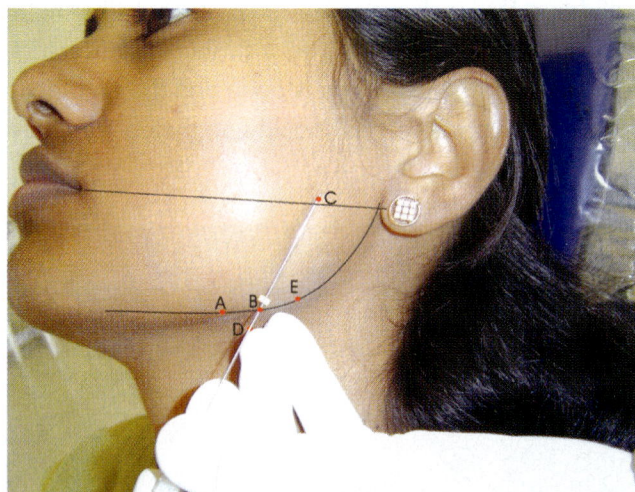

Fig. 9-3B: Needle is placed on the face parallel to the posterior border of the ramus of mandible. This would be the direction of injection from the lower border of the mandible close to the inner surface of the mandible. For injection a separate sterile needle is used

the lower border of the mandible, 3 mm below point 'B'. The needle when inserted should be kept parallel to the posterior border of ramus of mandible and inserted up to the rubber stopper.

10 Premedication and Sedative Techniques

Sedating a patient before local anesthesia is sometimes required in patients who are extremely nervous, non-co-operative children and mentally retarded individuals. Premedication refers to administration of drugs before a dental procedure to reduce anxiety, fear and apprehension. Some of the drugs used for premedication might be habit-forming and it is best to avoid use of such drugs. Premedication in children should be used with caution as the drug response is completely unpredictable. Routine use of premedication in every patient should be avoided. The value of preoperative counseling is more beneficial than routine use of premedication. Patient-doctor relationship plays an important role in allaying anxiety especially in children. A dental practitioner who is in constant contact and conversation with the patient and his family is in a better position to convince a patient to undergo dental procedures without fear or anxiety. When there is lack of personal touch, communication and pleasant approach, the patients do get apprehensive. This is especially true in case of children.

OBJECTIVES OF PREMEDICATION

- To reduce anxiety and fear
- To produce amnesia
- To decrease secretions
- To aid in induction of anesthesia
- To decrease the amount of anesthetic required.
- To decrease the possible toxic reaction to local anesthetics
- To decrease reflex excitability.

ROUTES OF DRUG ADMINISTRATION

Oral Route

The drugs to be administered by this route are usually dispensed in the tablets, capsules, and syrup form. This is considered as a safe route, easily accepted by patients and is more economical. However, the effectiveness of administration of drugs through oral route depends upon the amount of drug absorbed through the GI tract which is highly unreliable. There could be gastric irritation, nausea, vomiting and can also result in overdosage. Allergic reactions may also be encountered.

Intramuscular Route

This involves injecting the drug into the substance of the muscle which is not so easily acceptable as the oral route. However, a patient would prefer an im injection to intraoral injection. Although the onset of action is slow it is more predictable. Irritation to the GI tract is totally eliminated. Disadvantage is fear of injection and presence of pain.

The action of drugs administered by im or oral route in children is unpredictable. Elderly patients are increasingly sensitive and hence dosage might have to be reduced. Healthy adults might require additional dosage for a tranquilizing effect. The dosage when properly calculated and administered should give fairly acceptable results in managing anxiety and fear towards dental treatment.

Intravenous Route

Sedation by intravenous technique is the safest method where the dosage can be titrated. Conscious sedation implies that the patient is sedated to a level of consciousness in which he is able to maintain a patent airway independently and should respond to oral commands or to physical stimulation during the procedure. The drugs used to produce this state should possess a wide margin of safety, that is between conscious and unconscious state. Unless the drug is carefully titrated the patient may very quickly drift into unconsciousness. Since most of the dental procedures involve handling of tissue in the oral cavity, situation might get complicated if the patient drifts into unconscious state. Here the maintenance of airway becomes highly important. Airway management in case of children requires special considerations because of narrow nasal passages, glottis with hypertrophic tonsils or increased secretions. Conscious sedation by iv route in dental office is undertaken in western countries in clinics which are well equipped and by dental surgeons who have undergone special training in anesthesia. In India intravenous sedation is not undertaken in private dental clinics. It is wise to do these procedures in a hospital or a nursing home with the help of a trained anesthetist. There is no programs in India for dental surgeons to undergo training in anesthetic techniques.

DRUGS USED FOR PREMEDICATION BY ORAL AND IM ROUTE

1. Benzodiazipines
2. Narcotics
3. Miscellaneous

Benzodiazipines

These drugs produce tranquilization and controls anxiety. They do not cause sleepiness or hangover. They have skeletal muscle relaxation properties and act as anticonvulsants. The drugs in use are:

1. Diazepam
2. Midozolan
3. Lorazepam

Diazepam

This tranquilizing drug causes certain amount of amnesia along with muscular relaxation. The patient is usually alert and cooperative. Since the drug has no analgesic properties, proper local anesthetic should be administered before undertaking dental procedures. The drug when administered via oral route, achieves blood level within 2 hours. For dental outpatients 5 mg tablets can be given the night before and 5 mg 1 hour before the dental procedure. The unpredictability of its absorption from GI tract should be borne in mind. Intramuscular injections can also be used 1 hour before the procedure. For im use, 10 mg injections can be given.

Midozolan

It has similar tranquilizing action as diazepam but three times more potent. It can be administered intramuscularly and has quick onset of action. It is also eliminated rapidly. It has a better sedative and more amnesic effect. Dosage for im use is 0.1 to 0.15 mg/ kg body weight. Its use is not recommended for patients below 18 year of age.

Lorazepam

This can be classified as a sedative hypnotic. When administered the night before it gives an undisturbed sleep and relaxes the patient for the dental procedure the following day. The drug has a short half-life and carries no hangover effect. It can be administered in 1.5 mg.

Narcotics

These groups of drugs have more analgesic properties and reduces overall anesthetic requirement. The main drawback to the use of narcotic drugs is their effect of postoperative nausea and vomiting. The commonly used drugs are pentozocine, meperidine and Fentanyl.

Meperidine: This is a water soluble synthetic opiate, which can be administered by submucosal and im route.

Dosage is 1 to 2.2 mg / kg body weight. It should not exceed 100 mg.

Fentanyl: This synthetic derivative is a potent analgesic. It can be administered by im or submucosal route. It is used in dosage of 0.002 to 0.004 mg / kg body weight.

Miscellaneous

Chloral Hydrate and Trichlorphos: This group of drug act as sedative, hypnotic and also has antihistaminic properties. They are stable and less irritating. Trichlorphos is an ester of trichlorethonol which has similar properties as chloral hydrate. Chloral hydrate is available in capsule or elixir form. It is given in dosage of 500 to 1000 mg at bedtime. Trichlorphos is available an elixir in 0.5 g / ml. It can be administered in 50 to 70 mg / kg body weight.

INTRAVENOUS SEDATION

The advent of intravenous sedation for ambulatory patients in dental office has been an important advancement in the management of pain and anxiety. The primary concern is the safety associated with using potent drugs via the iv route.

Sedative anesthesia techniques from the hospital operation area to dental office, without proper preparation are fraught with potential complications. Many differences are present between the two techniques. One of the major difference between hospital and dental office anesthesia is the control of respiration. In the hospital the airway and respiration is closely monitored and oxygen is always available to supplement respiration. In majority of dental offices patient intubation is rarely undertaken. In the absence of endotracheal anesthesia the patient is at greater risk of aspiration and hypoxia. Again in the absence of intubation the patency of airway is wholly depended upon physical maintenance of the lower jaw and tongue in a forward position. Apart from this the anesthetist and the surgeon have to prevent any foreign objects from obstructing the airway.

The aim of conscious sedation is to achieve a satisfactory relaxation and cooperation without

compromising of vital functions. There is no definite amount of dosage and the drug has to be titrated slowly in each individual to avoid precipitious effect on cardiopulmonary and CNS.

Drugs for IV Sedation

Diazepam

Diazepam is quite popularly used for premedication in dentistry. Diazepam has quick onset of action. It reduces anxiety and the patients feel relaxed. There might be slight drowsiness but the patient is usually alert. As the drug has no analgesic properties local anesthesia has to be administered. The dosage for intravenous use varies from 10 to 20 mg in a healthy adult. As diazepam causes local irritation at the site of injection and possible thrombophlebitis, a lipid emulsion (Diazenulus) is used. The emulsion is less irritant and the possible occurrence of thrombophlebitis can be avoided. While administering the drug, should there be overdosage, airway patency should be ensured and simultaneously 100% oxygen should be administered.

Midozolam Hydrochloride

This drug can also be used for intravenous sedation. The drug is three times more potent that diazepam and is less irritant at the site of injection. The effective dosage is 0.1 mg / kg body weight and for conscious sedation 0.05 to 0.07 mg / kg body weight. As elderly patients are sensitive the drug dosage in such cases should be reduced. Midozolam produces certain amount of dose related antiretrograde amnesia. In higher doses it produces some respiratory depression.

Meperidine Hydrochloride (Pethidine)

Pethidine has a sedative analgesic and atropine-like effect. It is advantageous to use pethidine along with pentobarbitol since it prevents vomiting sensation symptoms of meperidine and also has an amnesic and analgesic effect without loss of consciousness. The effective dosage of pethidine is 0.25 to 1 mg / kg body weight and for conscious sedation ranges from 12.5 to 50 mg. The drug is contraindicated in patients known to be allergic and also in patients who are taking monoamine oxidase (depressant) inhibitors.

Petazocine Hydrochloride

This is a narcotic analgesic which has both agonistic and weak antagonistic properties. Conscious sedation can be achieved with 0.2 to 0.5 mg/kg body weight. Disadvantage of the drug is its high incidence of unwanted effects – including hallucinations, nightmares, dizziness, nausea and vomiting.

Fentanyl

This is highly lipid soluble synthetic opioid which has quick acting short duration of action. It is 100 times more potent than morphine. Conscious sedation is achieved with a dosage of 0.5 to 1 microgram / kg body weight. Fentanyl and its congeners like Alfentanyl citrate, Sufentanyl citrate have little or no effect on cardiovascular system. The adverse effects of these agents are typical of all opioids including dose dependent respiratory depression, skeletal muscle rigidity, occasional bradycardia, nausea and vomiting.

It is important to asertain patient's medical history and recording of vital signs such as pulse, BP and respiratory rate. Each patient must be queried in depth to evaluate the present state of health, past medical history, medications taken, allergies and drug reactions. Medical opinion should be sought when required.

Monitoring

The following equipments should be available to monitor the patient during the time the patient is under the influence of intravenous medication.

1. Electrocardiogram
2. Pulse oximetry for recording oxygen saturation.

In addition rate of respiration should be monitored. Equipments like laryngoscope (Fig. 10-1), endotracheal tubes (Figs 10-2A and B), airways (Fig. 10-4), mask

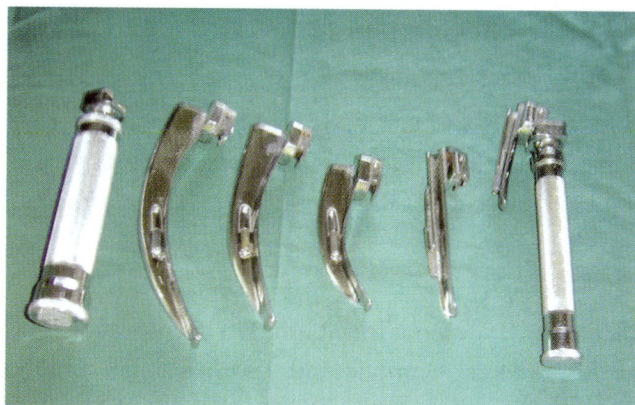
Fig. 10-1: Laryngoscope with different attachments

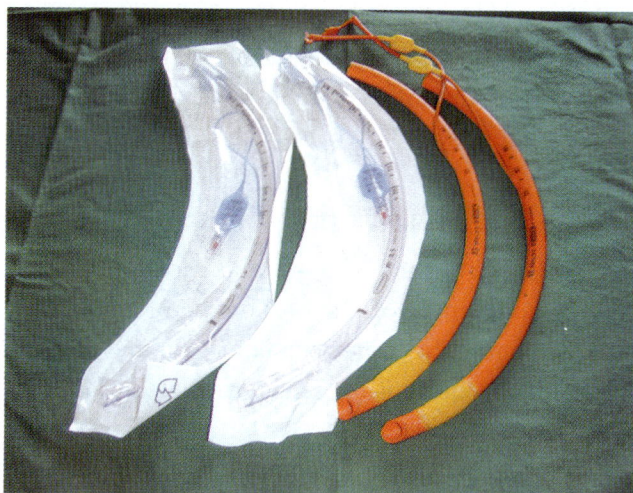
Fig.10-2A: Adult endotracheal tubes—Rubber and PVC disposable rubber tubes were being used repeatedly after sterilization. They are no more in use

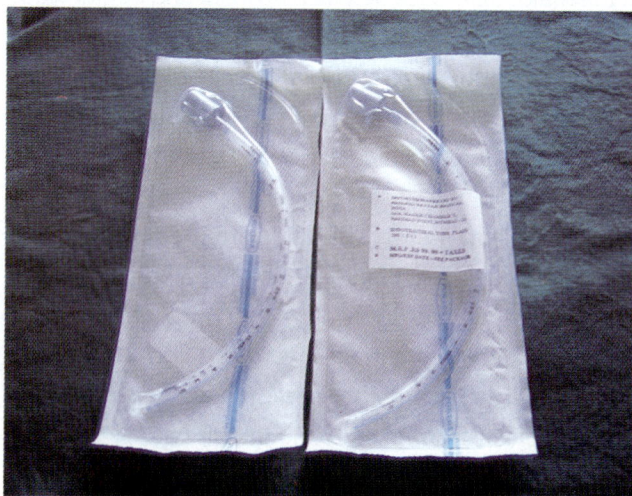
Fig.10-2B: Disposable endotracheal tubes—Pediatric

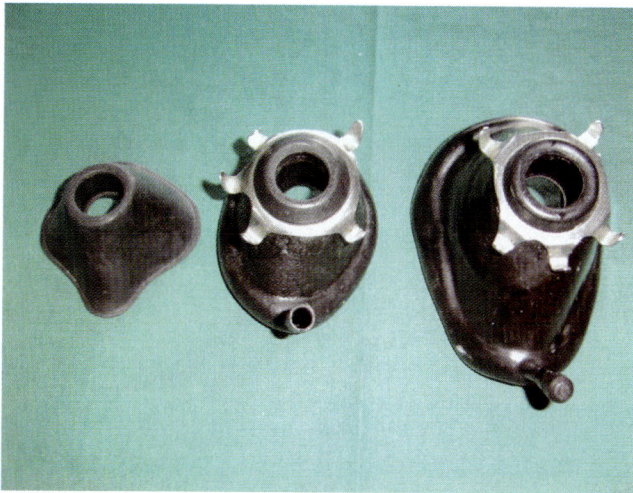

Fig. 10-3: Masks—For adults and children

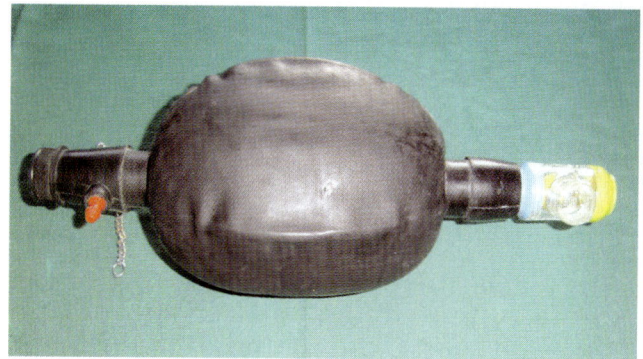

Fig. 10-5: Ambu bag

(Fig. 10-3), ambu bag (Fig. 10-5) and oxygen should be readily available. Emergency drugs like adrenaline, atropine, sodabicarb, calcium gluconate and few antiarrhythmic drugs like xylocard, dilzem should be stored for ready use.

Points to Remember Regarding Narcotics

1. Narcotic analgesics have profound effect on respiration.
2. Most of the narcotics are primarily indicated to provide analgesia.
3. It is difficult to titrate the narcotics.

4. Narcotics produce a fair incidence of nausea and vomiting.
5. All narcotics produce histamine release.
6. Narcotics are invariably used as part of the multidrug regimen.

Complications of Intravenous Sedation

1. Complications of venipuncture.
2. Complications due to adverse drug reactions and interactions.
3. Complications secondary to underlying medical illness.

Technique of Venipuncture

For safe administration of the drug it is necessary to establish a intravenous drip of saline or dextroase. An intravenous cannula is used for insertion into the vein. The vein in the cubital fossa is usually selected for venipuncture. After successfully positioning, the needle is inserted into the vein, the tubing is properly taped and secured. The selected drug is injected slowly through the open line.

Figures 10.6 to 10.10 shows the steps in venipuncture.

Complications of Venipuncture

Hematoma formation is the common complication where the blood leaks into the interstitial tissues. This results in immediate swelling and later echymosis of the

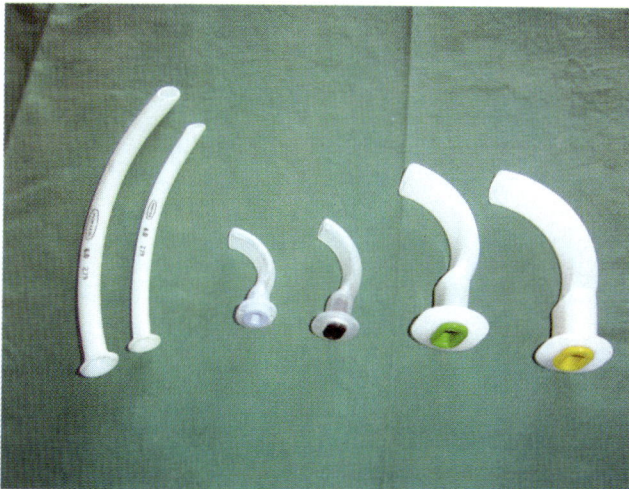

Fig. 10-4: Pharyngeal airways

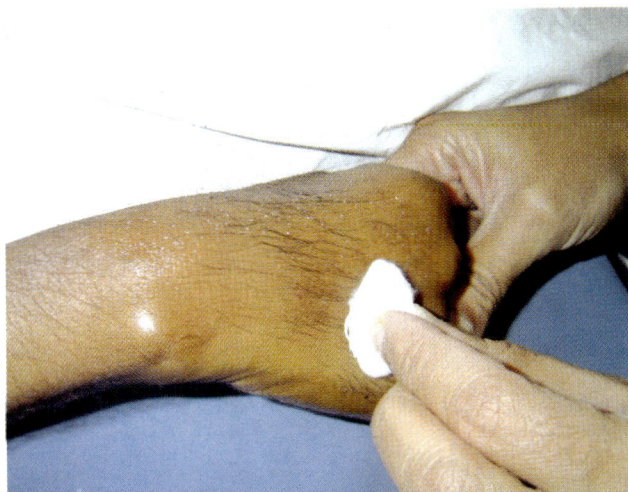

Fig. 10-6: Surface of the back of hand being disinfected by wiping with betadine antiseptic solution before venipuncture

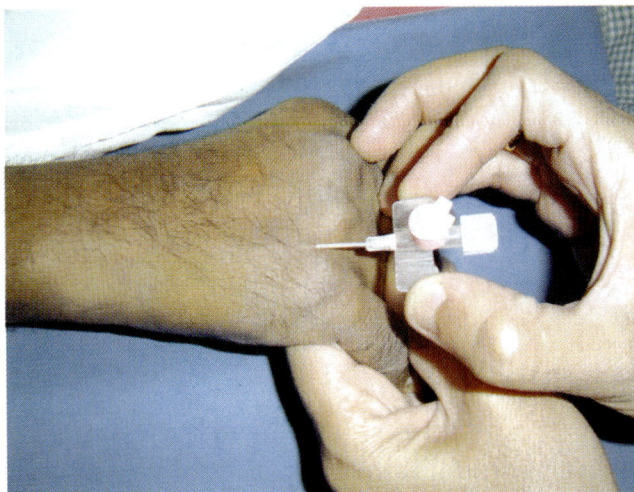

Fig. 10-8: Intravenous cannula being introduced into the vein

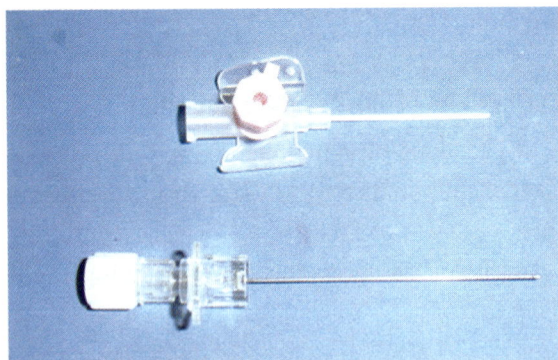

Fig. 10-7: Intravenous cannula

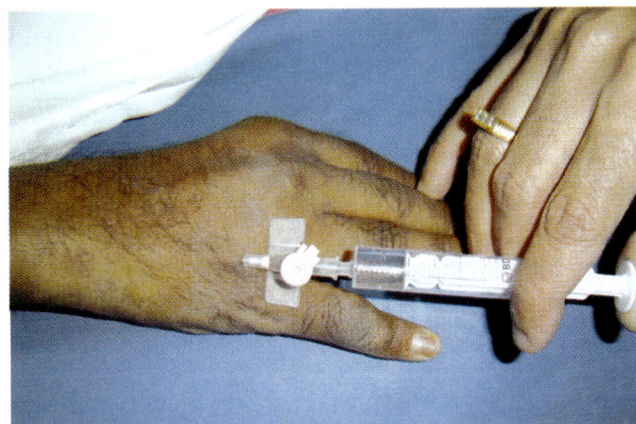

Fig. 10-9: Normal saline being flushed through the cannula

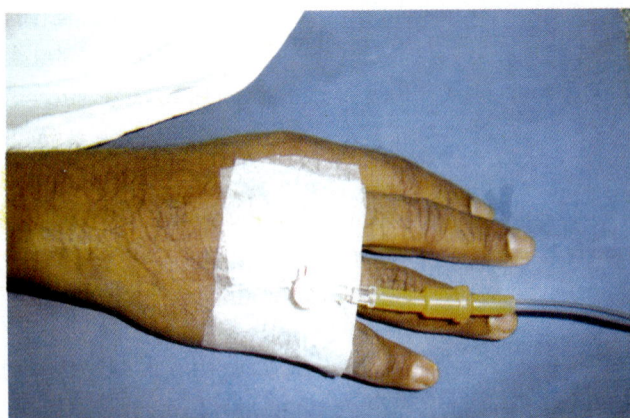

Fig. 10-10: Intravenous line is connected with the cannula well secured into place

area. If pressure is applied immediately the swelling can be minimized.

Vasospasm is due to local irritation which causes burning sensation in the area. This usually subsides after a few minutes and can be minimized by flushing the line with saline.

Phlebothrombosis results due to needle injury or drug irritation. This is often seen in hospitalized patients receiving fluids for a lengthy period. A localized swelling appears which is tender on palpation, usually resolves after application of hot compresses. This complication is commonly seen with diazepam injections.

Hypersensitivity and drug interactions can occur with any of the drugs. Since there will an open line through the skin, they can be effectively controlled by use of emergency drugs.

11

Complications of Local Anesthesia

Complications arising subsequent to injections of local anesthetic agents are fairly common. Most of the complications are minor in nature and can be treated without much difficulty. To effectively manage the complications, one should have a thorough knowledge of anatomy, innervation of the region, properties of anesthetic agents and proper techniques of administration. By strict observance of standard precautions many of the complications can be totally prevented.

Complications due to local anesthetics can be broadly classified as *immediate* and *late complications* (Table 11.1).

Table 11-1: Complications of local anesthestics

I. *Immediate complications*
   a. Pain during injection
   b. Burning sensation during injection
   c. Breakage of needles
   d. Syncope
   e. Hematoma
   f. Toxic reactions
   g. Allergic reactions
   h. Anesthesia in non-specific regions
 II. *Late complications*
   a. Self-inflicted trauma
   b. Infections
   c. Difficulty in opening of the mouth
   d. Paresthesia

IMMEDIATE COMPLICATIONS

Pain During Injection

Each patient reacts differently to injections in the oral cavity. Psychologically patients do not accept intraoral injection to be less painful; infact the sight of a syringe with needle, instruments and equipment itself make them apprehensive. Intraoral injection could be more acceptable if patients are briefed and assured before the surgical procedure. Children could be totally unpredictable. Some of them are very cooperative and the rest are just the opposite. Educating the children regarding anesthesia and the benefits of treatment will help in gaining their confidence. Engaging the child in general conversation will be helpful in future co-operation. Syringe, needle, instruments should be kept away from the patient's direct vision. Sometimes if the treatment is not urgent, it should be taken up after a few casual visits of the child to the dental office.

Pain during needle insertion could be avoided or minimized with the application of topical anesthetic agents at the area of injections. Many patients are so much used to this application of topical anesthesia before injections; they make a request for such application during subsequent injections.

Pain is also experienced during deposition of solution if it is carried out at a rapid pace; especially during palatal injections. This pain can be effectively controlled if the deposition of the solution is done slowly. Normally one full minute should be taken to deposit 2 ml of solution.

Usage of 25 to 27 gauge needles is preferred in dental practice. Thick gauge needles do cause certain amount of pain during insertion, and the sight of the same makes the patient slightly uncomfortable. Assurance to the patient that a fine gauge needle is being used goes a long way in securing the patient's co-operation.

During inferior alveolar nerve block, the needle sometimes may pierce the nerve. This results in a sudden shocking pain. In this situation the needle should be withdrawn for about 2 mm and the solution can be deposited. The pain in these cases is not possible to avoid as this is accidental and is very rare. The patient should be informed of the cause of pain. The needle injury in these cases, on rare occasions might result in prolonged post-injection anesthesia.

Burning Sensation during Injection

Burning sensation during deposition of anesthetic solution can occur:

1. When the anesthetic solution is contaminated.
2. When the cartridges stored in cold sterilizing solutions are used.
3. When alcohol is not used to wipe the rubber diaphragm of the cartridge or multidose vials.
4. When needle is inserted in areas where antiseptic solution has been applied.

These complications can be prevented by the following precautionary measures.

1. All discolored solution and anesthetic drug beyond expiry date should be discarded.
2. The preservation of anesthetic cartridges in cold sterilizing solution is not required. The rubber diaphragm of the cartridge or the multidose vial can be easily sterilized by wiping the area with ethyl alcohol. It is important to wait for the alcohol to evaporate failing which the needle will be contaminated with alcohol.
3. Application of antiseptic solution in the area of needle insertion is a standard practice. One should not forget to wipe off the remaining antiseptic solution from the area with sterile gauze. This will prevent contamination of the needle with the antiseptic solution.

Breakage of Needle

In today's modern dental practice there is total awareness of cross-infection and fear of HIV infections. This has resulted in widespread use of disposable syringes and needles. Thenceforth, breakage of needles during injections is almost nil. Although several cases of breakage of needles have been reported in dental literature, such incidences are not common in India. Infact the author has come across just 2 cases of needle breakage in the last 35 years of dental practice. This may be due to the fact that the use of cartridge syringes with 27 to 30 gauge needle was being used by very few dental surgeons and that too for a short period. Infact at present, there are very few manufacturers of anesthetic cartridges in India. In the beginning there was wide usage of glass syringes with 1½ inch, 22 to 24 gauge needles. The use of cartridges was not very popular due to cost factor. Then came the era of disposable syringes.

Needle breakage used to occur when the same needle was repeatedly sterilized and used in number of patients. The needle breakage is usually at the junction of the needle and the hub or at the point where it is bent and straightened. The dictum during insertion of needle is that it should not be inserted into the tissues more than ¾ of its length. It may be said that the needle breakage is entirely due to negligence on the part of the operator. Use of very fine gauge needle, for example, 30 gauge needle may result in breakage in case of the sudden movement of the patient. It is prudent to use short needles for infiltration and longer needles for block anesthesia.

When there is needle breakage, it is important not to panic and ask the patient to keep the mouth open. If the needle is visible at the site of needle puncture, it can be easily removed with the help of a mosquito hemostat. If the tip is not seen, the position of the needle should be localized by proper X-ray and the patient should be referred to a maxillofacial surgeon. In this situation it is important to inform the patient and assure that no complication will arise. Although opinions vary on the removal of broken needle, it is the author's opinion that a careful dissection should be made and the broken part of the needle should be removed. Leaving the needle in the tissue might cause psychological fear in the patient's mind and might also lead to litigation.

Syncope

Syncope or fainting is one of the most common complication occurring in dental office. This reaction is entirely due to psychogenic stress, upright position of the chair during injections, fright at the sight of syringe, needle, instruments and equipment along with possible fear of pain. The psychological fear factor triggers a vasovagal attack. There will be vasodilatation of the peripheral vessels and reduction of the heart rate, reducing the blood flow to the brain. This results in cerebral ischemia, which causes fainting. Vasodilatory effect occurs due to reflex stimulation of vasodilatory center at the anterior hypothalamus. Reduction in heart rate occurs due to stimulation of the vagal centers of the medulla. Because of the vasodilatory effect and the upright position of the patient the blood pools in peripheral and splanchnic vessels.

Although fainting is not a serious complication if not properly treated, could result in loss of consciousness, respiratory and cardiovascular depression. Before fainting, the patient exhibits certain symptoms and if the operator is observant, it can be prevented by simple measures. The pallor of mucous membrane, tongue, and face are early signs, which should be noted by the operator. If unattended to, there will be sweating, shivering, rolling of eyes and nausea. Sometimes there could be sudden convulsions followed by fainting. The patient will be unresponsive. When fainting occurs, the patient should immediately be placed in a reclining position with legs placed at a higher level than the head. The patient should be encouraged or coaxed to breathe deeply through his nose while the mouth is kept closed. The neck should be slightly extended to facilitate easy breathing. In a situation where the patient is seated in an ordinary chair, the patient should be assisted in bending forward with the head between the knees. This may not be possible in obese and pregnant women. In such situations, the patient should be immediately shifted and placed on the floor. With these few simple measures, usually the patient recovers and most of the time nothing more needs to be done. Syncope can be totally prevented if the patient is placed in a semi-reclining position in a physiological dental chair during administration of local anesthesia. In India, many dental surgeons have been performing dental procedures in a sitting position with the patient in reclining position, but many operators still use the standing position with the patient in upright position. It is also important to keep the patient in the semi-reclining position even after his recovery. If the patient is feeling fit, the concerned procedure can be carried out in the same position. If the patient is feeling very weak, it is better to postpone the procedure to a future date with proper preoperative preparation.

Hematoma

During intraoral injections, especially during block anesthesia, there are chances of the needle puncturing a blood vessel, resulting in blood accumulation in the tissues. This is more likely to occur during tuberosity or infraorbital block. In either instance there is a sudden development of swelling due to accumulation of blood in the tissues. During inferior alveolar nerve block, rarely injury occurs to superficial vessels, which sometimes results in submucosal hemorrhage. The swelling due to hematoma may result in difficulty in opening of the mouth and chewing. When the swelling starts to appear, hand pressure over the swelling is applied for about 15 minutes. This results in compression of the tissues and thereby the vessels, which usually stops the internal bleeding and further increasing of swelling. Application of cold packs also prevents further increase of swelling as it causes vasoconstriction in that region.

The patient should be explained the reason for the swelling and be assured that the swelling will reduce on its own within a few days time. After 48 hours, warm applications can be applied which hastens the process of phagocytosis of the broken down red cells from the tissues.

Toxic Reactions

Toxicity of a drug is usually related to overdosage and rapid absorption of the anesthetic solution, which results in the presence of high concentration of the drug in the blood circulation. This can result in depression of the central nervous system (CNS) and the cardiovascular system (CVS). Under the normal circumstances with the use of therapeutic dose of anesthetic solution, it causes little or no untoward effect on CNS or CVS. The anesthetic solution, apart from its action on nerve endings gets absorbed into blood circulation. The absorption of anesthetic solution into circulatory systems depends upon the vascularity of the area and the presence or absence of vasoconstrictor in the anesthetic solution. When an anesthetic agent is used without vasoconstrictor, the absorption into circulation would be faster and moreover, the anesthetic agents in general have a vasodilatory action. The addition of a vasoconstrictor to an anesthetic solution causes constriction of blood vessels and reduces the rate of absorption from the tissues.

The anesthetic drug in the blood undergoes bio-transformation and ultimate elimination. The site of biotransformation varies with different groups of agents. In case of ester group of agents, the biotransformation occurs in the blood. In case of amide group of agents, the bio-transformation is almost entirely in the liver. Finally the anesthetic agents are all excreted through the kidneys. This process of absorption, hydrolization and excretion is a continuous process. Toxic reactions occur when there is a sudden increase in blood concentration of the anesthetic agent, which may occur in case of accidental direct injection of the anesthetic solution into a blood vessel. Toxic blood level may also appear in cases where a large volume of anesthetic solution is injected due to unsatisfactory anesthesia.

The toxic level of anesthetic agent affects all exicitable tissues especially CNS and CVS. Initially there will be cerebral stimulation followed by medullary depression. The initial clinical manifestation of CNS toxicity results in convulsive episode. There could be shivering and twitching of muscles in general. The patient may feel dizzy and get totally disoriented. This initial reaction is followed by depression. In case of amide group of anesthetic agents, the first reaction could be that of sedation. This toxic manifestation usually is transitory as the anesthetic agent in circulation is being continuously hydrolyzed and removed from the system.

Toxic effect of local anesthetic agents on the CVS is that of depression. It depresses the heart rate and reduces the blood pressure and respiratory rate. With the usage of normal amount of anesthetic solution the blood concentration is about 0.5 to 2 mg/ml. This concentration has absolutely no effect on CNS or CVS. The clinical manifestation of toxicity is observed only in cases where the blood level of the anesthetic agent rises to 6 mg/ml of blood. It is extremely rare that the toxic reaction will lead to severe respiratory depression and subsequent cardiac arrest. However, one should be well versed with remedial measures to be undertaken under such an event. A good knowledge of method of resuscitation of a patient, who has gone in for a cardiac arrest is mandatory (refer cardiac resuscitation).

Mild toxic reactions are most of the time transitory and no treatment is indicated. The patient usually recovers in a few minutes time. In severe toxic reactions the patient should be protected from further injury during convulsions. Medical help should be immediately sought. Airway patency should be ensured by slightly lifting up the neck in reclining position. Oxygen, if available, should be administered. If oxygen is not available, patient should be instructed to take deep breath through the nose while keeping the mouth closed. Pulse rate and blood pressure should be monitored. Convulsions can be managed by administration of anticonvulsant drugs such as thiopentone (150-250 mg iv) or diazepam (10-20 mg iv). Profound hypotension should be treated by injection of atropine (0.5 to 1.5 mg iv). Occasionally adrenaline can be used to control the bradycardia.

Toxic reaction resulting from overdosage can be easily prevented. Most of the procedures in dental practice do not require more than 4 to 6 ml of 2% lidocaine with adrenaline. If an operator is injecting beyond 6 ml of anesthetic solution to obtain a satisfactory anesthesia, it should be assumed that the procedure of anesthetic injection is not proper. Aspirating the syringe each time before the solution is deposited will prevent the accidental intravascular injection.

Allergic Reactions

Allergic reactions to local anesthetic agents could be 'localized' or 'systemic' in nature. Local reactions, though are annoying can be easily treated. Systemic anaphylactoid type of reaction should be managed properly, failing which it can lead to fatality. Paraminobenzoic acid group of derivatives are known to cause allergic reactions but from the time the amide group of anesthetic agents have been in usage, the allergic reactions are rare. Sometimes some of the constituents of the anesthetic solution may give rise to allergic reactions. Methylparaben and propylparaben which are used as antibacterial and preservative are found to have given rise to allergic reactions. These two preservatives are used in multidose vials. The use of parabens in anesthetic cartridges have been discontinued in USA since 1982. The anesthetic derivatives manufactured in India at present are packed in multidose vials, containing methylparaben as preservative. Use of cartridges in India was for a brief period. At present very few dental surgeons use cartridges. This may be because of the high cost of cartridges and also that of cartridge syringes. At present the disposable syringes and needles are used by majority of dental surgeons.

Mild allergic reactions can manifest in the form of itching, skin rashes and angioneurotic edema. In severe cases, there can be anaphylactoid type of reaction, which can result in dyspnea, cyanosis, peripheral vascular collapse and ultimately death. A person with a history of allergy, branchial asthma, allergic rhinitis, nasal polyps and skin disorders has to be carefully evaluated.

The details of previous dental intervention, occurrence of any untoward reactions, and patient's records would give an idea of susceptibility of the person. There is every likelihood of the condition being confused for syncope. A patient sometimes may not know the type of anesthetic agent used in his previous treatment. In the absence of records, it is difficult to know which derivative of anesthetic he is allergic. In all these cases it is better to investigate the susceptibility of the patient. This can be carried out by a simple procedure. 0.2 ml of the anesthetic solution (to be used) should be injected intradermally on the forearm of the hand. The area of insertion is marked with a circle with a marking pen. After 30 minutes if there is urticaria, edema or redness of the area within the circle it should be assumed that the patient is allergic to that particular anesthetic drug. Sometimes even this small dose of anesthetic agent can trigger anaphylactoid type of reaction. Since there are number of laboratories for testing allergy to various agents, it is safer to refer the patient to such centers.

Mild allergic reactions, to anesthetic solutions can be managed by use of antihistaminic drugs. Administration of diphenhydramine (benadryl) 25-50 mg 3 to 4 times for 2 to 3 days or pheniramine maleate 25 mg 2 to 3 time for 2 or 3 days should effectively control the histamine type of allergic reaction.

In case of severe allergic reactions, apart from skin reaction and smooth muscle spasms, even respiratory and cardiovascular involvements are prominent. Clinically the patient feels sick with vomiting and itching sensation. Flushing of the face and subconjunctival hemmorrhage can be noted. Because of the smooth muscle spasms, there could be fecal and urinary incontinence. Simultaneously, due to edema of pharyngeal region there will be wheezing, dyspnea, hypertension, cyanosis leading to unconsciousness and finally cardiac arrest. Any negligence in recognition and execution of planned appropriate treatment, the patient might die within 5 to 10 minutes.

Management

The patient should be positioned comfortably in semireclining position. Bronchodilators in the form of aerosol spray should be administered, following which medical assistance should be sought immediately. 100% oxygen should be administered. Simultaneously 0.3 to 0.5 mg of epinephrine should be injected by iv route. 20 to 50 mg of diphenhydramine should be administered im or iv. 100 mg of hydrocortisone sodium succinate should be given im or iv. Epinephrine should be repeated every 5 minutes depending upon the condition of the patient. By this time if the patient's airway is not clear, crycothyrotomy should be performed.

Apart from this monitoring the vital signs are most important. If the patient does not improve within five minutes of administration of first injection of epinephrine, the patient may go in for cardiac arrest. One should be ready to institute cardiopulmonary resuscitation (refer resuscitation).

Anesthesia in Nonspecific Regions

Anesthesia occurring in undesired places is totally due to wrong technique of administration of local anesthetic injections. In case of inferior alveolar nerve block, the needle sometimes may be inserted too far back of the ramus resulting in deposition of anesthetic solution in the parotid gland. This leads to anesthesia of facial nerve resulting in temporary Bell's palsy. If the landmarks for the block are properly observed and the syringe is kept in proper direction, this complication should not occur. Moreover if the needle insertion is more than 1 inch into the tissues, then one should assume that the direction of the needle is not proper. To reach the parotid gland one should insert the full length of 1½ inch needle, which is total negligence on the part of the operator.

LATE COMPLICATIONS

Lip Trauma

The effect of anesthesia from an inferior alveolar nerve block lasts for nearly 2 to 2½ hours. During this period, if the patient has not been properly instructed in post-operative care, the person may injure himself by biting on the lip, cheek or tongue and may also scald the lip or cheek while consuming hot beverages. As the area is totally anesthetized, the patient is unaware of the injury and hence the patient should be made aware of this complication and should be instructed not to eat or drink hot beverages till the anesthesia wears away completely. This complication can be more common in children if proper care is not taken.

Infections

Infection following intraoral injections can occur only if the needle and syringe are not properly sterilized. Use of contaminated anesthetic solution can also result in post-injection infections. With the usage of disposable needles and syringes, the chances of infection from this source is nil. Repeated insertion of the rubber diaphragm of anesthetic multidose vials may also result in contamination of the solution. It is prudent to use a thicker gauge needle, e.g. 22 gauge needle, to aspirate the solution from the vial and a finer needle can be used for injection of the solution into the tissues. The thicker needle can be left in the vial and stored in a sterile area for further use.

Difficulty in Opening the Mouth

Difficulty in opening the mouth is commonly refered to as 'trismus'. This occurs due to unintended damage to the muscle fibers of medial pterygoid muscle during inferior alveolar nerve block. The trismus is due to reflexive spasm of the muscle. Sometimes trismus may also result from hematoma formation in the pterygoid space or in the retromolar region. Very rarely does trismus occur due to infection from the needle or contaminated anesthetic solution.

Management consists of warm mouth rinsing coupled with jaw opening exercises. Administration of 50 mg of diclofenac with paracetamol 500 mg tablets will relieve pain and inflammation. Improvement in opening of the mouth may not be immediate but will get better in about a week's time. In cases of post-injection infection, appropriate antibiotics should be administered.

The muscle damage by the needle results, only if needles are repeatedly used after sterilization. This can be prevented by using disposable needles.

Paresthesia

This is a subjective sensation, which could be anesthesia, hypo- or hypersensation, which is experienced by the patient in the form of numbness, tingling, or pin-pricking sensation. The causative factor is injury to the nerve fibers, which occurs during anesthetic injections or during surgery. Pressure from blood clot or an impacted tooth impinging on the nerve can also result in paresthesia. Normal sensation usually returns but may take anywhere between 2 to 6 weeks of time. It is important to reassure the patient regarding the recovery of the sensation.

CARDIOPULMONARY RESUSCITATION (CPR)

Cardiac arrest in dental practice is extremely rare. However in case a patient goes in for a cardiac arrest it is highly important that every dental surgeon should be in a position to perform CPR. It is necessary that every practicing dental surgeon should undergo training in the method of CPR. All the emergency drugs should be available in easy reach and the containers should be boldly marked for easy identification. Updating on the step-by-step procedure and the dosages, time to time is essential. This will enable a dental surgeon to perform this life saving procedure in times of emergency.

Procedure of CPR

If the patient is unconscious he should be placed on a firm flat surface. The contour dental chair can be placed in a horizontal position (Fig. 11-1). Head should be tilted up, to clear the airway (Figs 11-2 and 11-3). If necessary the mandible can be held forward. Summon medical help. Feel for the carotid pulse (Fig. 11-4). If the pulse is not felt inject adrenaline (epinephrine) 0.3 ml of 1:1000 intravenously. If it is not possible to inject iv, im injection should be done immediately without delay. Check the breathing by placing you cheek close to the nose. Introduce an oropharyngeal airway.

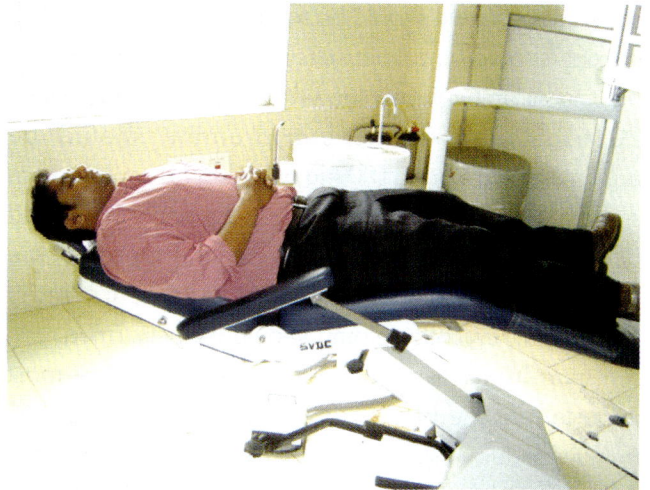

Fig. 11-1: Patient being placed in a horizontal position

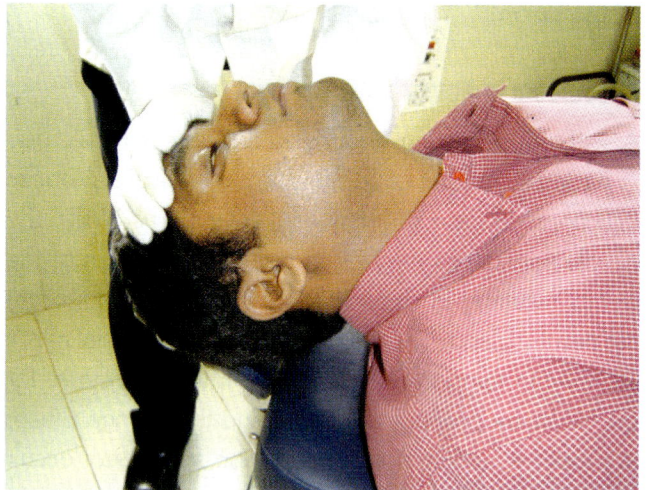

Fig. 11-2: Head being tilted to clear the airway

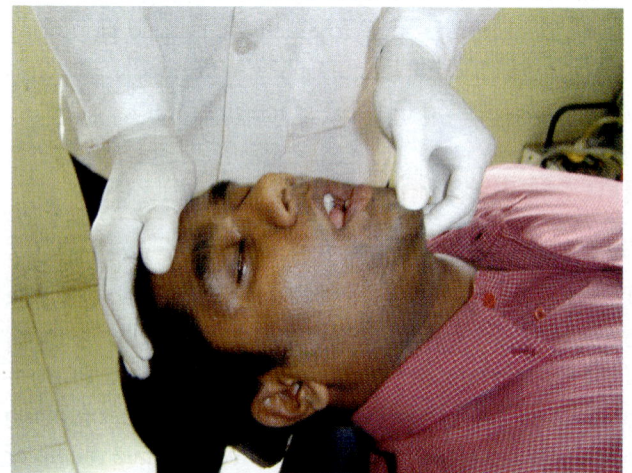

Fig. 11-3: Mandible being pushed forward in open mouth position

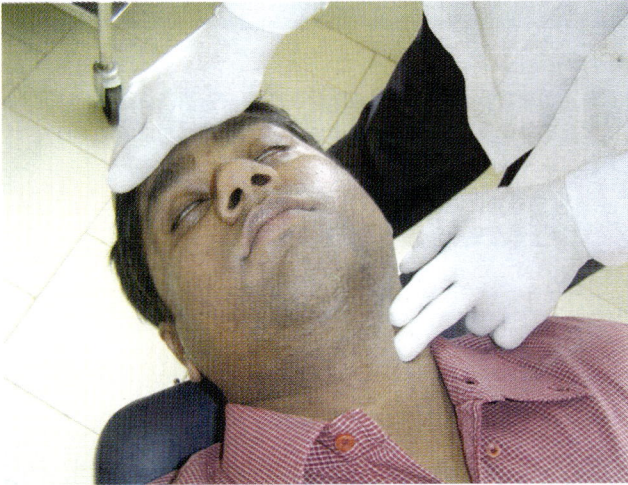

Fig. 11-4: Carotid pulse being felt

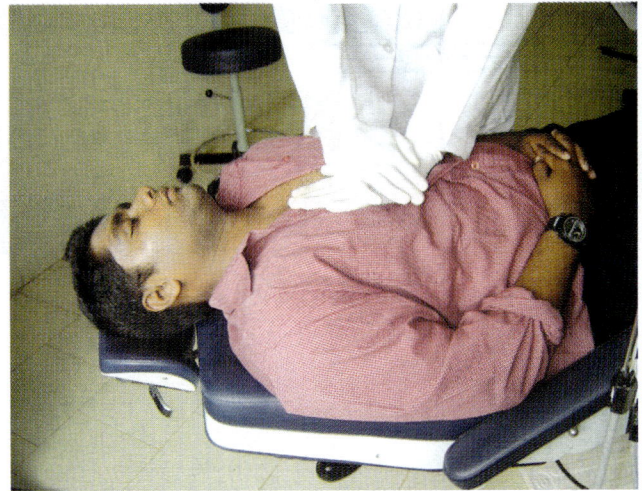

Fig. 11-6: Alternative placement of hand and fingers for external cardiac massage

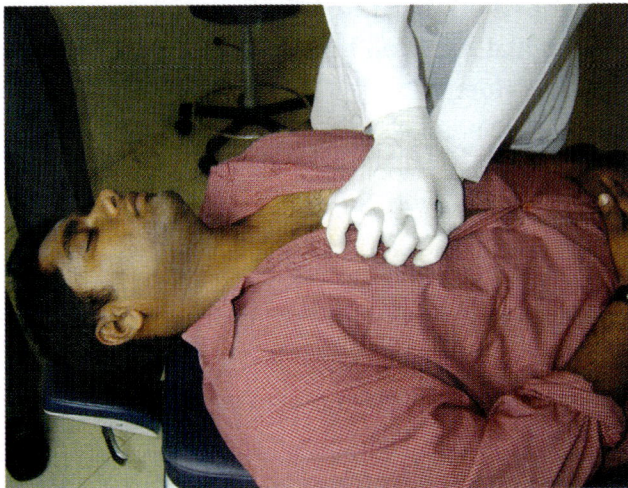

Fig. 11-5: Position of the operator for external cardiac massage

External cardiac massage should be started immediately. If the patient is placed on the floor the doctor should kneel by the side of the patient. Place the heel of the left hand over the sternum at its lower 1/3

position. The right hand is placed over the back of the left hand and the fingers are interlocked (Figs 11-5 and 11-6). The arms are kept straight. The compression should be done using the force from the shoulder area without bending. The compressions should be 60 to 90 / minute. The sternum should be compressed 2 inches every second. If single-handed then the person should alternate five compressions with one forced mouth-to-mouth or mouth-to-nose breathing. The forced breathing can also be carried out through a pharyngeal airway. When mouth-to-mouth breathing is being carried out nose must be pinched close by fingers. If an assistant is present one person can handle cardiac compression while the other does the forceful breathing. Regular assessment of the patient's condition should be done by feeling for the pulse and observing the color of the patient's face. This may have to be continued till medical help arrives.

Multiple Choice Questions in Local Anesthesia

1. **To extract the first maxillary molar the following nerves should be anesthetized:**
   1. Nasopalatine nerve
   2. Anterior palatine nerve
   3. Posterior palatine nerve
   4. Anterior superior alveolar nerve
   5. Middle superior alveolar nerve
   6. Posterior superior alveolar nerve
   A. 1, 5, 6
   B. 2, 4, 5
   C. 2, 5, 6
   D. 3, 5, 6

2. **Which of the following block anesthesia procedure most likely to result in hematoma:**
   A. Mental nerve block
   B. Infraorbital nerve block
   C. Inferior alveolar nerve block
   D. Posterior superior alveolar nerve block

3. **Lip biting self injury is a post-injection complication of:**
   A. Posterior superior alveolar nerve block
   B. Inferior alveolar nerve block
   C. Infraorbital nerve block
   D. Anterior palatine nerve block

4. **Paresthesia of the lip results in:**
   A. Numbness in the area
   B. Hypersensitive reaction in the area
   C. Hypoesthesia in the area
   D. Tingling sensation in the area
   E. All of the above

5. **Which of the following mandibular teeth causes slight pain during extraction after anesthetizing the inferior alveolar nerve, lingual nerve and the long buccal nerves on one side:**
   A. Canine tooth
   B. 3rd molar tooth
   C. Central incisor
   D. Premolar teeth

6. **Allergy to anesthetic solution may be due to:**
   A. Procaine hydrochloride
   B. Adrenaline which is used as vasoconstrictor
   C. Methylparaben
   D. Propylparaben
   E. All of the above

7. **The initial toxic reaction to xylocaine injection is:**
   A. Twitching of muscles
   B. Shivering
   C. Talkativeness of the patient
   D. Sleepy feeling

8. **Which condition amongst the following, use of local anesthetic is contraindicated:**
   A. 3rd month of pregnancy
   B. Patient on dialysis
   C. Cirrhosis of liver
   D. Hypersensitivity to the anesthetic drug

9. **Hematoma resulting during posterior superior alveolar nerve block injection is due to:**
   1. Needle injury to posterior superior alveolar blood vessels
   2. Injury to pterygoid plexus of veins
   3. Injury to internal maxillary artery
   4. Injury to temporal branch of facial artery
   A. 1, 2
   B. 2, 4
   C. 1, 3
   D. 1, 2, 4

10. **Which of the following causes toxic reaction due to overdosage:**
    A. Rapid absorption of anesthetic solution
    B. Use of large volume of anesthetic solution
    C. Accidental intravenous injection of anesthetic solution
    D. Delayed excretion of the drug due to cirrhosis of the liver
    E. All of the above

11. **Needle breakage during injections is most likely to occur due to:**
    A. Sudden movement of patient during injection
    B. Repeated sterilization and use of the same needle
    C. During intraligamentary injection
    D. Use of fine gauge needle in intracanalicular injections
    E. All of the above

12. **Paresthesia of lower lip may result due to:**
    A. Mandibular radicular cyst
    B. Malunited fracture of mandible in the parasymphysis region
    C. Surgical removal of lower impacted 3rd molar
    D. Extraoral mandibular nerve anesthesia

13. **Infiltration anesthesia is not effective in the first molar region in the maxilla due to:**
    1. Presence of thick alveolar bone at the root of zygoma
    2. Absence of porous bone in the 1st molar tooth region
    3. Dual nerve supply to the mesio buccal root
    4. Presence of three roots
    A. 1, 3
    B. 1, 2
    C. 3, 4

14. **Trismus resulting after inferior alveolar nerve injection is most likely due to:**
    A. Hematoma formation
    B. Damage to medial pterygoid muscle fibers
    C. Injection into parotid gland
    D. Injury to the mandibular nerve

15. **Lignocaine hydrochloride is:**
    A. A basic compound
    B. An amide derivative
    C. An ester derivative
    D. An aldehyde

16. **Syncope occurring in dental office is due to:**
    A. Temporary cerebral anemia
    B. Use of vasoconstrictors in local anesthetic solution
    C. Injury to nerve during injection of local anesthetic solution
    D. Allergic reactions

17. **Which of the following maxillary teeth is difficult to anesthetize by infiltration anesthesia:**
    A. Maxillary canine
    B. Maxillary third molar
    C. Maxillary central incisor
    D. Maxillary first molar

18. **To achieve maxillary nerve anesthesia the anesthetic solution should be deposited in the:**
    A. Infraorbital foramen
    B. Foramen ovale
    C. Nasopalatine canal
    D. Greater palatine foramen

19. **Earliest sign of syncope is:**
    A. Pallor of face, tongue and mucous membrane
    B. Sweating
    C. Rapid breathing
    D. Vomiting sensation

20. **Injury to inferior alveolar nerve during nerve block injection can result in:**
    A. Permanent anesthesia in the lower lip region
    B. Temporary paresthesia of the lower lip
    C. Inability to close the lips
    D. Temporary anesthesia of anterior 2/3 of tongue
    E. Difficulty in speech

21. **In Gow Gates technique the anesthetic solution is deposited :**
    A. At the mandibular fossa
    B. At the foramen ovale
    C. At the anterior region of condyle
    D. In the pterygomaxillary space

22. **Maximum dosage of 2% Lignocaine with 1:1,00,000 Epinephrine in a healthy adult is:**
    A. 4.4 mg / kg   body weight
    B. 6.6 mg / kg   body weight
    C. 7.0 mg / kg   body weight
    D. 3.5 mg / kg   body weight

23. **Which of the following agents could be effectively used for topical anesthesia:**
    A. Mepivacaine
    B. Procaine
    C. Prilocaine
    D. Benzocaine

24. **Methemoglobinemia occurs in patients receiving large doses of :**
    A. Procaine
    B. Lignocaine
    C. Prilocaine
    D. Bupivacaine

25. **Majority of local anesthetic preparations without the addition of a vasoconstrictor have a pH of:**
    A. 5.5
    B. 6.0
    C. 6.5
    D. 7.0

26. **The pH of tissue fluids is around :**
    A. 5.5   B. 6.8
    C. 7.0   D. 7.4

27. **To prolong the local anesthesia and to obtain profound anesthesia:**
    A. Repeat injection should be given when the patient is still under local anesthetic effect
    B. Repeat injection should be given few seconds after the patient feels the pain
    C. Repeat injection should be given few minutes after the patient feels slight pain

28. **Hydrolysis of Procaine anesthetic drug takes place:**
    A. Almost entirely in Plasma
    B. Almost entirely in Liver
    C. 60% occurs in plasma and 40% in Liver
    D. Major portion in plasma

29. **Toxic dosage of lignocaine for a pediatric patient occurs at:**
    A. 2.2 mg / kg body weight
    B. 4.4 mg / kg body weight
    C. 2.4 mg / kg body weight
    D. 2.1 mg / kg body weight

30. **Which of the following statement is false:**
    A. Syncope is also termed as fainting
    B. Syncope is transient reversible loss of consciousness
    C. Syncope results from altered circulation
    D. Syncope is due to angina attack

31. **In which of the following condition infiltration anesthesia is differed:**
    A. Infection
    B. Renal failure
    C. Patient under dialysis
    D. All the above

32. **In a resting state the nerve membrane is:**
    A. Slightly permeable to Na^+ ions
    B. Not permeable to Na^+ ions
    C. Permeable to Na^+ ions depending upon the concentration of K^+ ions
    D. It is freely permeable to Na^+ ions

33. **During repolarisation:**
    A. Excess of Na ions moves out of the nerve tissue passively
    B. Excess of Na ions are removed via the sodium pump
    C. Removal of Na ions depends upon the concentration of K^+ ions

34. **Conduction of impulse in myelinated nerve fiberes—which of the following is true:**
    A. Is slow due to thick myelin sheath
    B. Continuous conduction of nerve impulse occurs along the core axoplasm
    C. Due to saltatory effect the conduction is faster

35. **Administration of bilateral inferior alveolar nerve block:**
    A. Is contraindicated since the tongue might fall back and obstruct the airway
    B. Is contraindicated since it may result in difficulty in swallowing
    C. Is contraindicated as the patient may aspirate
    D. Is not contraindicated

36. **Inferior alveolar nerve block injection without proper sterilization might result in primary infection of the:**
    A. Pterygomandibular space
    B. Buccal space
    C. Massetric space
    D. Temporal space

37. **Lidocaine as local anesthetic is preferred to procaine:**
    A. Since it causes less depression of CNS
    B. Since it causes less cardiovascular collapse
    C. Since it causes less incidence of allergic reactions
    D. Since it is 50% more potent than procaine

38. **Which of the following anesthetic derivatives produces significant stimulation of cerebral cortex :**
    A. Cocaine
    B. Lidocaine
    C. Procaine
    D. Tetracaine

39. **In severe trismus of the jaw the following intraoral technique is followed to anesthetize inferior alveolar nerve :**
    A. Clark and Holmes technique
    B. Sunder Vajirani technique
    C. Gow Gates technique
    D. Classic inferior alveolar nerve block.

40. **Which of the following local anesthetic solution causes vasoconstriction without the addition of a vasoconstrictor:**
    A. Cocaine
    B. Lidocaine
    C. Procaine
    D. Bupivacaine

41. **Administration of Local anesthesia is contraindicated in case of:**
    A. Hypertension
    B. Diabetes mellitus
    C. Thyrotoxicosis
    D. Anemia
    E. All of the above

42. **With anesthesia of inferior alveolar nerve and lingual nerve which of the following teeth could be removed without pain:**
    A. All molars
    B. All teeth on that half of lower jaw

C. Premolars and molars

D. Premolars and anterior teeth

E. Premolars, lateral incisor and canine

43. During administration of inferior alveolar nerve block the following muscle is pierced by the needle:

A. Temporalis

B. Superior constrictor muscle of pharynx

C. Masseter

D. Buccinator

44. Of the action of Epinephrine, which of the following is not true:

A. It produces increase in blood pressure

B. Produces dilatation of coronary arteries

C. Constricts smaller blood vessels

D. Decreases incidence of dysarrhythmias

45. Average duration of nerve block anesthesia with 2% lignocaine + 1:200,000 epinephrine lasts:

A. More than 60 minutes

B. Less than 60 minutes

C. Less than 30 minutes

D. More than 120 minutes

46. Local anesthetic injections results in loss of function in which order?

1. Touch

2. Temperature

3. Proprioception

4. Pain

5. Skeletal muscle tone

A. 1, 2, 3, 4, 5

B. 4, 2, 1, 3, 5

C. 2, 5, 4, 1, 3

D. 5, 3, 4, 2, 1

47. Following repolarization, the recovery of functions is in which order?

1. Touch

2. Temperature

3. Proprioception

4. Pain

5. Skeletal muscle tone

A. 1, 2, 3, 4, 5

B. 2, 1, 4, 3, 5

C. 5, 3, 1, 2, 4

D. 5, 4, 1, 2, 3

48. To attain loss of function which of the following does not require higher concentration of anesthetic:

A. Pain

B. Motor nerve

C. Heat

D. Cold

E. Pressure

49. In development of adequate anesthetic concentration in the nerve fibers which of the following factor influences the same:

A. Too high or too low tissue pH

B. Excessive dilution with blood or tissue fluids

C. Too rapid absorption of the anesthetic into the systemic circulation

D. Use of vasoconstrictors in the anesthetic solution

50. Which of the following does not result in toxic overdosage:

A. Use of too large dose of anesthetic solution

B. Unusual rapid absorption of the anesthetic solution

C. Unintentional intravenous injection of the anesthetic solution

D. Unusual slow biotransformation

F. Use of an anesthetic drug with adrenaline

51. Which of the following is not a sign when there is toxic reaction to overdosage of local anesthetic on CNS:

A. Talkativeness

B. Sweating

C. Muscular twitching

D. Dizziness

E. Light headedness

G. Flushing of the face

52. **Which of the following symptoms of allergic reaction to local anesthetic drug does not occur:**
    A. Rashes
    B. Urticaria
    C. Angioneurotic edema
    D. Muscle twitching and tremors
    E. Nasal congestion

53. **Which of the following treatment is not indicated in cases of allergic reaction to anesthetic solution:**
    A. Antihistamine agents
    B. Epinephrine inhalants
    C. Antiemetics
    D. Epinephrine (0.5 ml of 1:1000 im)
    E. Aminophyline (0.5 mg iv)
    F. Oxygen

54. **The following are the features of general anesthesia *except*:**
    A. Loss of sensation
    B. Unconsciousness
    C. Muscle relaxation
    D. Abolition of reflexes
    E. Hypothermia

55. **Horace Wells who invented Nitrous oxide was:**
    A. A Dentist
    B. A Lawyer
    C. An Engineer
    D. A Doctor
    E. A Scientist

56. **Guedel described 4 stages of anesthesia with:**
    A. Halothane
    B. Chloroform
    C. Isoflorane
    D. Ether

57. **Colour of Nitrous oxide cylinder is:**
    A. White
    B. Blue
    C. Orange
    D. Black
    E. Green

58. **Oxygen content in atmospheric air is:**
    A. 21%   B.   30%
    C. 50%   D.   65%
    E. 79%

59. **Which drug is called white stuff in anesthesia practice:**
    A. Thiopentone sodium
    B. Cocaine
    C. Propofol
    D. Chloroform
    E. Ketamine

60. **The following are benzodiazepines *except*:**
    A. Diazepam   B. Lorazepam
    C. Midazolam   D. Pentazocine
    E. Clonazepam

61. **The aims of preanesthesia medication are all of the following *except*:**
    A. Relief of anxiety
    B. Amnesia
    C. Decreases secretions
    D. Analgesic action
    E. Unconsciousness

62. **All of the following are muscle relaxants *except*:**
    A. Succinylcholine
    B. Pancuronium
    C. Fentanyl
    D. Atracurium
    E. Vecuronium

63. **All of the following are true regarding thiopentone *except*:**
    A. Used in induction of anesthesia
    B. Anticonvulsant

C. Short acting

D. Used in narco analysis

64. **The dose of midazolam used for conscious sedation is:**
    A. 0.01 mg / kg body weight
    B. 0.1 mg / kg body weight
    C. 0.5 mg / kg body weight
    D. 1 mg / kg body weight
    E. 2 mg / kg body weight

65. **Oral airway is used for all except:**
    A. Protection of airway
    B. Prevent tongue falling back
    C. Prevent tongue bite
    D. Prevent aspiration

66. **All of the following inhalational agents are liquids except:**
    A. Ether
    B. Desflurane
    C. Isoflurane
    D. Nitrous oxide
    E. Enflurane

67. **Atropine used during anesthesia in all of the following except:**
    A. Anti-sialogogue action
    B. During bradycardia
    C. Heart block
    D. Tachycardia

68. **The drug used to reverse neuromuscular paralysis is:**
    A. Atropine
    B. Neostigmine
    C. Naloxone
    D. Glylopyrrolate
    E. Adrenaline

69. **For nasotracheal intubation which of the following tubes are used:**
    A. Ryle's tube
    B. Segstaken tube

C. Endotracheal tube

D. None of the above

E. All of the above

70. **Laryngoscope is used for all of the following except:**
    A. Direct visualisation of larynx
    B. For endotracheal intubation
    C. For insertion of Ryle's tube
    D. Pharyngeal airway

71. **ASA in anesthesia means:**
    A. American Society of Anesthesiologists
    B. Asian Society of Anesthesiologists
    C. African Society of Anesthesiologists
    D. Australian Society of Anesthesiologists
    E. None of the above

72. **In severe liver disease which of the following anesthetic drug can be safely used:**
    A. Procaine
    B. Lidocaine
    C. Mepivacaine
    D. Prilocaine

73. **In a known case of allergy to procaine which of the following anesthetic would be contraindicated:**
    A. Topical spray of Tetracaine
    B. Topical spray of Lidocaine
    C. Injection of Mepivacaine
    D. Injection of Prilocaine

74. **Bupivacaine is derivative of:**
    A. Para-amino benzoic acid
    B. Xylidine
    C. Toluidine
    D. Anilide

75. **How much lidocaine is present in a dental cartridge (1.8 cc) containing 2% Lidocaine with 1: 100,000 adrenaline:**
    A. 36 mg per cartridge

B. 25 mg per cartridge

C. 30 mg per cartridge

D. 28 mg per cartridge

76. **How much epinephrine is present in a dental cartridge (1.8 cc) containing 2% Lidocaine with 1: 100,000 epinephrine:**
   A. 0.01 mg per cartridge
   B. 0.018 mg per cartridge
   C. 0.05 mg per cartridge
   D. 0.012 mg per cartridge

77. **As per the specific receptor theory which of the following is true:**
   A. Decreases the permeability of the nerve membrane to sodium ions
   B. Decreases the conduction of potassium ions through the nerve membrane
   C. Increases the sodium ion permeability
   D. Facilitates binding of calcium ions

78. **Which of the following anesthetics has the highest lipid solubility:**
   A. Procaine   **B.** Mepivacaine
   C. Bupivacaine   **D.** Lidocaine

79. **Which of the following anesthetic drug bonds with the protein for a longer duration:**
   A. Procaine   **B.** Bupivacaine
   C. Lidocaine   **D.** Prilocaine

80. **The administration of local anesthetic in normal accepted dosage to a pregnant woman will affect the healthy child:**
   A. True
   B. False

81. **If you inject an anesthetic solution with Pka value of 8.1 into tissue with pH of 7.4; what amount of the drug would be ionized in the tissues:**
   A. Over 50%
   B. At 50%
   C. Below 50%

82. **Who invented Ethyl ether:**
   A. Horace Wells
   B. WTG Morton
   C. JY Simpson

83. **In which stage of general anesthesia excitement is characterized:**
   A. Stage – I   **B.** Stage – II
   C. Stage – III   **D.** Stage – IV

84. **Which of the one is not true of Nitrous oxide:**
   A. It is non-inflammable gas
   B. It has high patient acceptability
   C. It is a highly potent anesthetic
   D. It produces analgesia at 65% concentration

85. **Which of the one is not true of Halothane:**
   A. It is not explosive
   B. It is highly potent
   C. It is irritating to mucous membrane
   D. It produces incomplete muscle relaxation
   E. It tends to produce hypotension
   F. It sensitizes heart to epinephrine

86. **Who synthesized procaine in 1905:**
   A. Niemann
   B. Koller
   C. Halstead
   B. Einhorn

87. **Who gave the first inferior alveolar nerve block anesthesia by using 4% cocaine:**
   A. Niemann
   B. Horace Wells
   C. Einhorn
   D. Halstead

88. **Which is the convenient stage of general anesthesia when surgery can be performed:**
   A. Stage – I
   B. Stage – II
   C. Stage – III
   D. Stage – IV

89. To achieve hemostasis in a surgical area which of the following is anesthetic preparation is recommended:
A. 2% Lidocaine HCl without vasoconstrictor
B. 2% Lidocaine HCl with 1: 50,000 epinephrine
C. 2% Lidocaine HCl with 1:100,000 epinephrine
D. 2% Lidocaine HCl with 1:200,000 epinephrine

90. To achieve deep general anesthesia:
A. Percentage of oxygen to be increased
B. Do not extend the neck after inducement
C. By administring adrenaline i.v
D. Achieve higher alveolar concentration of anesthetic agent

91. Pain sensation is conducted through:
A. A alpha fibers
B. A gamma fibers
C. A beta fibers
D. A delta fibers

92. A woman in her late pregnancy should never be placed in the supine position in dental chair because:
1. It can produce caval compression
2. The uterus may press on inferior vena cava
3. It can produce hypotensive syndrome
A. 1 and 2
B. 1 and 3
C. 2 and 3
D. 1, 2 and 3

93. A few minutes after inferior alveolar nerve block patient develops paralysis of muscles of forehead, eyelids and lower lip on the same side because of anesthesia of branches of:
A. Otic ganglion
B. Facial nerve in the parotid gland
C. Ophthalmic branch of trigeminal nerve
D. Motor branch of the mandibular nerve

94. Local anesthetic agent acts on:
A. Nerve membrane

B. Myelin sheath
C. Axoplasm
D. Perineurium

95. Which of the following is contraindicated in a patient with glaucoma:
A. Xylocaine
B. Epinephrine
C. Phenobarbitone
D. Atropine

96. Which of the following is not fast pain:
A. Sharp pain
B. Pricking pain
C. Acute pain
D. Throbbing pain

97. Which of the following is not slow pain:
A. Burning pain
B. Aching pain
C. Electric pain
D. Chronic pain

98. By which route of administration a drug will have a definate predictable response:
A. Intramuscular
B. Oral
C. Subcutaneous
D. Intravenous

99. To counteract the stimulation of CNS subsequent to accidental intravascular injection of anesthetic solution, which of the following drugs can be administered:
A. Adrenaline
B. Antihistamine
C. Pentobarbital
D. None of the above

100. Syncope can be effectively managed by:
A. Administration of 100% oxygen
B. Administration of antihistaminics
C. Lowering the head position below the level of feet
D. By placing the patient in recovery position

101. **For cardiac massage to be effective, the sternum should be depressed:**
   A. 2 inches every second
   B. 3 inches every second
   C. 2 inches every 5 seconds
   D. 3 inches every 5 seconds

102. **An instant swelling appearing on the side of face immediately following a posterior superior alveolar nerve block anesthesia is most probably due to:**
   A. Drug allergy
   B. Infection
   C. Injury to blood vessel
   D. Intravascular injection

103. **Which of the following drugs used for premedication cause hallucination:**
   A. Midazolam hydrochloride
   B. Fentanyl
   C. Diazepam
   D. Pentozocine hydrochloride

104. **Which of the following is not a standard anesthetic cartridge available:**
   A. Cartridge with 1.8 ml
   B. Cartridge with 1.7 ml
   C. Cartridge with 2 ml
   D. Cartridge with 2.5 ml

105. **Premedication is administered to:**
   A. Reduce anxiety
   B. Produce amnesia
   C. Decrease reflex excitability
   D. Decrease secretions
   E. All of the above

106. **Local anesthetic drugs are metabolized or hydrolyzed in:**
   1. Plasma
   2. Liver
   3. Lungs
   A. All of the above   B. 1 and 2
   C. 1 and 3   D. None of the above

107. **During inferior alveolar nerve block the needle passes through:**
   A. Mucous membrane, areolar tissue, fat and masseter muscle
   B. Mucous membrane, buccinator muscle and areolar tissue
   C. Mucous membrane, areolar tissue and medial pterygoid muscle
   D. Mucous membrane, superior constrictor muscle of pharynx and areolar tissue

108. **Common complication encountered subsequent to anesthetic injection in a dental office:**
   A. Syncope   B. Trismus
   C. Hematoma   D. Bell's palsy

109. **In hyperthyroidism patients, anesthetic drugs with adrenaline should not be used because it might cause**
   1. Increased sensitivity
   2. Toxic crisis
   3. Tachycardia
   4. Fainting
   5. Chest pain
   A. 1,2,4
   B. 2, 3, 5
   C. All of the above

110. **Threshold of pain tolerance is influenced by:**
   A. Fear and anxiety
   B. Mental status of the patient
   C. Age of the patient
   D. Previous experience
   E. All of the above

111. **Which of the following maxillary teeth require nerve block anesthesia for extracting the tooth:**
   A. Canine   B. Central incisor
   C. First premolar   D. First molar
   E. Second molar

112. **Syncope during anesthetic injection can be prevented by:**
    A. By administration of premedication
    B. By placing the patient in reclining position
    C. Aspirating the syringe before depositing solution
    D. All of the above

113. **Which of the following drugs result in least loss of reflexes:**
    A. Narcotics
    B. Halothane
    C. Thiopental
    D. Ether
    E. Nitrous oxide

114. **In which of the following conditions general anesthesia is contraindicated:**
    A. In a patient above 65 years of age
    B. In a diabetic patient
    C. In a patient with acute respiratory infection
    D. In a patient with a history of anginal attack
    E. In a patient with urinary infection

115. **During cardiac resuscitation which of the following indicates patient's recovery:**
    A. No change in sensorium
    B. Pupillary dilatation
    C. Pupillary constriction
    D. Increase in radial pulse rate

116. **If the response to syncope is ineffective and the condition of patient deteriorates which of the following you would carry out first:**
    A. Start intravenous line immediately
    B. Inject corticosteroids
    C. Inject adrenaline 1:1000 intravenously
    D. Administer 100% oxygen
    E. Start CPR

117. **Level of analgesia is best monitored by:**
    A. Heart rate
    B. Ocular movements
    C. Verbal response
    D. Muscle tone
    E. Respiration

118. **During syncope inhalation of amonia aromaticus acts as a:**
    A. Vasovagal stimulant
    B. Circulatory stimulant
    C. Respiratory stimulant
    D. Stimulation of first cranial nerve

119. **Accidental foreign body inhalation may land in:**
    A. Esophagus
    B. Left bronchus
    C. Right bronchus
    D. All of the above

120. **For effective anesthesia higher concentration of anesthetic solution is required in:**
    A. Myelinated nerve fibers
    B. Unmyelinated nerve fibers

121. **In which of the following, general anesthesia is contraindicated:**
    A. Allergic reactions to analgesic drugs
    B. Ophthalmic infections
    C. Severe anemia
    D. Urinary infections

122. **Effects of sedation can be reversed quickly during:**
    A. Intravenous sedation
    B. Oral route
    C. Inhalation
    D. Intramuscular

123. **Which of the following is true:**
    A. Prilocaine causes more vasodilatation than Mepivacaine
    B. Lidocaine causes more vasodilatation than Prilocaine
    C. Mepivacaine causes less vasodilatation than Lidocaine
    D. All of the above

124. **Benzocaine and Lidocaine base anesthetics for topical use are not soluble in:**
    A. Water
    B. Alcohol
    C. Glycol
    D. Polyethylene glycol

125. **Eutectic mixture of local anesthetics in a combination of:**

A. Lidocaine and Prilocaine

B. Lidocaine and Mepivacaine

C. Mepivacaine and Prilocaine

D. Prilocaine and Mepivacaine

ANSWERS

1 C	2 D	3 B	4 E	5 C	6 E	7 D	8 D
9 A	10 E	11 E	12 C	13 B	14 B	15 B	16 A
17 D	18 D	19 A	20 B	21 C	22 B	23 D	24 C
25 A	26 D	27 A	28 D	29 B	30 D	31 A	32 A
33 B	34 C	35 D	36 A	37 C	38 A	39 B	40 A
41 C	42 E	43 D	44 D	45 A	46 B	47 C	48 A
49 D	50 E	51 F	52 D	53 C	54 E	55 A	56 D
57 B	58 A	59 C	60 D	61 E	62 C	63 C	64 B
65 D	66 D	67 D	68 B	69 C	70 D	71 A	72 A
73 A	74 D	75 A	76 B	77 A	78 C	79 B	80 B
81 C	82 A	83 B	84 C	85 A	86 D	87 A	88 C
89 B	90 D	91 D	92 D	93 A	94 A	95 D	96 D
97 C	98 D	99 C	100 C	101 A	102 C	103 D	104 D
105 E	106 A	107 B	108 A	109 C	110 E	111 D	112 D
113 E	114 C	115 C	116 C	117 C	118 C	119 C	120 A
121 C	122 C	123 B	124 A	125 A			

Bibliography

1. Akinosi JO: A new approach to the mandibular nerve block. Br J Oral Surg 1977;15:83-87.
2. Aldrete JA, Johnson DA: Allergy to local anesthetics. JAMA 1969;207:356-57.
3. Arun B Samsi Rajaram A. Bhalerao, Sharad C Shah, Bimal Mody, Teresa Paul, Rajaninath S. Satorkar – Evaluation of Centbucridine as a local anesthetic. Anesth Analg 1983;62:109–11.
4. Astra Zeneca LP: EMLA drug information sheet, 2000.
5. Bartlett SZ: Clinical observations on the effects of injections of local anesthetics by, Aspiration, Oral Surg, Oral Med, Oral Pathol 1972;33:520.
6. Bennett CR: Monheim's Local Anesthesia and Pain Control in Dental Practice, St. Louis. The C.V. Mosby Co. 1974.
7. Blanton PL, Jeske AH : The key to profound local anesthesia: neuroanatomy. J Amer Dent Assoc 2003;134:753-60.
8. Brown OT, Beamish D, Wildsmith JA: Allergic reaction to an amide local anesthetic. Br J Anaesth 1981;53:435-37.
9. Campbell RL, Gregg JM, Levin KJ, et al: Vasovagal response during oral surgery. J Oral Surg 1976;34:690-700.
10. Clinicians guide to dental products and techniques. Septocaine. CRA Newsletter, June 2001.
11. Cowan A: Further clinical evaluation of Prilocaine (Citanest) with and without epinephrine, Oral Surg, Oral Med, Oral Pathol 1968;26:304-11.
12. Crose VW: Pain reduction in local anesthetic, evaluation of intracutaneous testing for investigation of allergy to local anesthetic agents. Anesth Analg 1970;49:173-81.
13. Frazer M: Contributing factors and symptoms of stress in dental practice. Br Dent J 1992;173(2):211.
14. Friedman MJ, Hochman MN: The AMSA injection: A new concept for local anesthesia of maxillary teeth using a computer controlled injection system. Quint Int 1998;29:297-303.
15. Friedman MJ, Hochman MN: 21st century computerized injection for local pain control, compend contin. Educ Dent 1997;8:995-1003.
16. Fukayama H, Yoshikawa F, Kohase H, et al: Efficacy of AMSA anesthesia using a new injection system, the Wand, Quint Int 2003;34:533-41.
17. Geoffrey LH, How, F.Ivor H.Whitehead : Local Anesthesia in Dentistry, (3rd edn), Wright, London.
18. Gibson RS, Allen K, Hutfless S, Beiraghi S: The wand vs. traditional injection: a comparison of pain related behaviours, Pediatric Dent 2000;22:458-462.
19. Goulet JP, Perusse R, Turcotte JY: Contraindications to vasoconstrictors in Dentistry: Part III, Pharmacologic Interactions, Oral Surg, Oral Med, Oral Pathol 1992;74(5):692-97.
20. Gow – Gates GAE : Mandibular conduction anesthesia : A new technique using extraoral landmarks, Oral Surg 1973;36:321-28.
21. Gupta PP, Tangri AN, Saxena RC, Dhawan BN: Clinical pharmacology studies on 4 – N – butylamino – 1, 2, 3, 4 – tetrahydroacridine hydrochloride (centbucridine)- a new local anesthetic agent. Indian J Exp Biol 1982;20:344-46.
22. Guyton AC : Basic Neuroscience: Anatomy and Physiology, Philadelphia: WB Saunders 1987.
23. Allen GD. Dental Anesthesia and Analgesia (3rd ed) CBS Publishers and distributors.
24. Hans Evers, Glenn Hugerstam – Introduction to Dental Local Anesthesia (2nd ed) Medi Globe SA, 1990.
25. Haas DA : An update on local anesthetics in dentistry, J Can Dent Assoc 2002;68:446-551.
26. Haas DA, Harper DG, Saso MA, Young ER: Comparison of Articaine and Prilocaine anesthesia by infiltration in maxillary and mandibular arches. Anesth Prog 1990;37:230-37.
27. Haas DA, Harper DG, Saso MA, Young ER: Lack of differential effect by Ultracaine (articaine HCL) and Citanest (Prilocaine HCL) in infiltration anesthesia, J Can Dent Assoc 1991;57:217-23.

28. Halstead CK, et al: Physical evaluation of the dental patient, St. Louis, The C.V. Mosby Co, 1982.
29. Harris WH, Cole DW, Mittal M, Laver MB: Methemoglobin formation and oxygen transport following intravenous regional anesthesia using Prilocaine. Anesthesiology 1968;29:65.
30. Hoffmann – Axthelm W: History of dentistry , Chicago, Quintessence, 339. 1981.
31. Inderbir Singh. Text book of Human Anatomy (4th ed). J.P Publishers, 1991.
32. Jackson D, Chen AH, Bennett CR: Identifying true lidocaine allergy. J Am Dent Assoc 1994;125 (10):1362-66.
33. Jaffe AS: The use of Antiarrhythmics in advanced cardiac life support. Ann Emerg Med 1993;22:307-16.
34. Knoll – Kohler E, Rupprecht S: Articaine for local anesthesia in dentistry: A lidocaine controlled double blind cross-over study. Eur J Pain 1992;13:59-63.
35. Kramer SL, Milton VA: Complications of local anesthesia. Dental Clin North Am 1973;17:443-60.
36. Malamed SF: Medical Emergencies in Dental Office (5th ed) St. Louis, Mosby, 1999.
37. Malamed SF: Handbook of Local Anesthesia (5th ed) Mosby Inc, 2004.
38. Malamed SF: Handbook of Medical Emergencies in the Dental office (ed.2) CV Mosby, St. Louis, 1982.
39. Margetis PM, Quarantillo EP, Lindberg RB: Jet injection local anesthesia in dentistry: A report of 66 cases, US Armed Forces Med, J 1958;9:625-34.
40. Melzack R, Wall PD: Pain mechanism: A new theory, Science 1965;150:971.
41. Monheim LM: Local Anesthesia and Pain Control in Dental Practice, (4th ed) St. Louis Mosby, 1969.
42. Moore PA: Preventing local anesthetic toxicity. J Am Dent Assoc 1992;123(3):60-64.
43. Moore PA: Bupivacaine a long- lasting local anesthetic for dentistry. Oral Surg 1984;58-369.
44. Moorthy AP, Moorthy SP, O'Neil R: A study of pH of dental local anesthetic solutions. Br Dent J 1984;157 (11):394-95.
45. Munshi AK, Hedge AM, Latha R: Use of EMLA: Is it an injection free alternative? J Clin Pediatr Dent 2001;25:215-19.
46. Nickel AA: Parasthesia resulting from local anesthetics. J Oral Maxillofac Surg 1984;42(5):279.
47. Naftalin LW, Yogiela JA: Vasoconstrictors: indications and precautions, Dent Clin N Amer 2002;46:433-46.
48. Norman Trieger – Pain Control (2nd ed) Mosby, 1994.
49. Patnaik GK, Dhawan BN: Pharmacological study of 4 – N – buty – lamino – 1, 2, 3, 4 – tetrahydroacridine hydrochloride (centbucridine) – a new local anesthetic agent. Indian J Exp Biol 1982; 20:330-33.
50. Patnaik GK, Rastogi SN, Anand N, Dhawan BN. Evaluation of local anesthetic activity of 4 – N – butylamino – 1, 2, 3, 4 – tetrahydroacridine hydrochloride (centbucridine) – a 4 substituted polymethylenequinoline. Indian J Exp Biol 1982;20:327–29.
51. Perry DA, Loomer PM: Maximizing pain control. The AMSA Injection can provide anesthesia with few injections and less pain. Dimensions Dent Hyg 2003;1:28-33.
52. Perusse R, Goulet JP, Turcotte JY: Contraindications to Vasoconstrictors in Dentistry: Part II. Hyperthyroidism, diabetes, sulfite sensitivity, cortico dependent asthma, and phenochromocytoma. Oral Surg 1992;74: 5687-91.
53. Robin A. Seymour, John G Meechan Michail S. Yates Pharmacology and Dental Therapeutics (3rd ed) Oxford University Press, 1999.
54. Rudolph H de Jong – Local Anesthetics, Mosby, 1994.
55. Richard S. Snell – Clinical Neuroanatomy for Medical Students (3rd ed) Little Brown and Company, 1992.
56. Seng GF, Gay BJ: Dangers of sulfites in dental local anesthetic solutions: Warnings and recommendations. J Am Dent Assoc 1986;113(5):769-70.
57. Sam V. Holroyd, Richard L. Wynn Barbara Requa – Clark Clinical Pharmacology in Dental Practice (4th ed) – CV Mosby Company, 1988.
58. Schulze – Husmann M: Experimental evaluation of the new local anesthetic. Ultracaine in Dental Practice (doctoral dissertation) Bonn, University of Bonn, 1974.
59. Schwartz HJ, Sher TH: Bisulfite sensitivity manifesting as allergy to local dental anesthesia. J Allergy Clin Immunal 1985;75(4):525-27.
60. Standards and guidelines for cardiopulmonary resuscitation (CPR) and emergency cardiac care (ECC), JAMA 1986;255:2905-89.
61. Steen PA, Michenfelder JD: Neurotoxicity of anesthetics. Anesthesiology 1979;50:437-53.
62. Sveen K: Effect of the addition of a vasoconstrictor to local anesthetic solution on operative and postoperative bleeding, analgesia and wound healing. Int J Oral Surg. 1979;8:301-06.
63. Saxena RC, Gupta PP, Sharma JN, Gupta NN, Dhawan BN: A clinical study with centbucridine, a new local anesthetic. Indian J Pharmacol 1973;5:244.
64. Saxena RC, Saxena SC, Agarwal KC: Centbucridine for surgical procedures. Indian J Pharmacol 1974;6:32.
65. Tripathy - Essentials of Medical Pharmacology (5th ed), J.P. Publishers, Delhi.
66. Van Eden SP, Patel MF: Prolonged parasthesia following inferior alveolar nerve block using Articaine. Br J Oral Maxilofac Surg 2002;40:519-20.

67. Van Oss GE, Vree TB, Baars AM, Termond EF, Booji LH : Pharmacokinetics, metabolism, and renal excretion of Articaine and its metabolite articainic acid in patients after epidural administration, Eur J Anaesthesiol 1989;6:19-56.

68. Vazirani SJ: Closed mouth mandibular nerve block: A new technique, Dent Dig 66:10-13,1960.

69. Vachrajani GN, Parikh, N, Paul T, Satorkar RS : A Comparative study of centbucridine and lidocaine in dental extraction. Int J Clin Pharmacol Res 1983;3(4):251–55.

70. Wolfe SH: The Wolfe nerve block: A modified high mandibular nerve block. Dent Today 1992;11:34-37.

71. Wilson AW, Deacock S, Downie IP, Zaki G: Allergy to local Anesthetic: the importance of thorough investigation. Br Dent J 2000;188:320-22.

72. Welden E Bell. Orofacial Pain (4 th ed) Year Book of medical Publishers.

Index